HEALING CAN
BE EASY

By Beth Misner, Ivan Misner, Ph.D., and
Betty Runkle, N.D. with Mohammad Nikkhah, D.C.

We dedicate this book to those who have given of themselves to teach and guide both of us along the path of natural healing: specifically to Betty Wells Runkle, N.D., and Dr. Mohammad Nikkhah, our coauthors; and additionally to Dr. Christian Issels, Dr. Walter Kim, Dr. Revel Miller, Dr. Isaí Castillo, Dr. Lise Janelle, Dr. Yolanda Arce, and Dr. Bill Kellas. In the areas of spiritual direction and inspiration to: Dawa Tarchin Phillips, Master Chunyi Lin, and Dr. Dawson Church. People like you selflessly help those of us who want to walk this path with the hope and confidence that healing naturally is possible.

Beth Misner and Ivan Misner, Ph.D.

I would like to dedicate this book first to my husband, Robert, who has supported me physically, mentally, and spiritually throughout the years of education and experimentation on my quests to find the most healthful and beneficial way of life for our family. And to my children, Ryan, Garrett, Jensyn, and Evan, who were so patient with me throughout the various transitions of our nutritional habits as I learned more and more how to lead and live a healthy, balanced lifestyle. Finally, to my father, Joe P. Wells, Ph.D., who instilled in me a love for learning and education and who taught me to appreciate science by definition: as a practical activity involving intellectual evaluation of systems, behaviors, and structures through observation and experimentation.

Betty Wells Runkle, N.D.

I would like to dedicate this book to my mother, Ashraf Beyzaei, and the memory of my father, Bagher Nikkhah.

Dr. Mohammad Nikkhah

PREFACE

I first met Beth and Ivan over ten years ago in the Transformational Leadership Council (TLC). I sensed immediately this beautiful couple were kind beings with a lot of love to share. They are open hearted, as well as open minded, and curious about the world I am constantly in, the world of qigong. Beth showed great interest in qigong (pronounced chee-gong), coming often to my Spring Forest Qigong (SFQ) morning classes held during our semi-annual TLC retreats. She has progressed to the point where she now leads the t'ai chi and qigong classes herself from time to time at the TLC conferences I do not attend.

Five years ago, when Beth and Ivan first asked me to work with them to help Ivan heal after his prostate cancer diagnosis, I was so grateful. Qigong is an ancient, scientifically based healing modality that is thousands of years old, and I help people discover their ability to transform energy on a daily basis. To be able to help my friends, Beth and Ivan, was a great pleasure for me.

And then to have Beth call me and share that she had discovered a small tumor in her body, even before she knew whether it was malignant or not, was also gratifying. I was so happy to be able to work with her to help her really understand how qigong healing works.

You see, qigong is the practice of working with energy (qi=energy, gong=work with), and everything in the universe is energy. This was understood by the ancient Chinese qigong masters, and it has been shown to be scientifically true by Albert Einstein, as well as other prominent scientists. What Beth was going to learn from her own experience was just how easily the body can heal when all the energy blockages are removed.

i

Illness comes about when there is a blockage in the normal flow of energy in our bodies. There are a variety of causes for energy blockages: injuries, emotions, stress, and infections, among other things. What Beth has learned during her time studying with me is that when the cause of the blockage is removed, her body's normal flow of energy is able to activate the innate healing capacity we all have within us.

Medical science now understands the vital importance of the BodyMind connection and interaction in health and wellness. What Western medicine still doesn't embrace fully is a simple, comprehensive way of enhancing this powerful connection; although a growing number of medical doctors are now recommending SFQ to their patients. Some of them, like the director of the Department of Integrative Medicine at the Mayo Clinic, have even personally requested that I contribute to a textbook for doctors and medical schools, which I have done.

Spring Forest Qigong is a proven system to enhance and optimize the connection between mind, body, and spirit in just minutes a day. In Beth's case, she practiced the SFQ Five Healing Elements three times each day! She worked with me and my team of qigong healers to create a qigong healing retreat for herself, joining us in Minneapolis, Minnesota, for nearly two weeks.

I am certain that her focus on opening energy blockages in her body is responsible for the speed at which her breast cancer was so easily healed. From the very beginning of her healing journey, she did the meditations and visualizations that have been effective for our SFQ students. She embraced the practice and the concepts of SFQ to use breathing, the power of the mind, movement, and sound to balance and enhance the flow of energy—Qi.

She understood from the beginning that the most powerful healing energy in the universe is unconditional love. She loved her body, and she even loved the cancer cells that were there to teach her a valuable lesson about life. She loved others around her, unconditionally, and she healed just as her husband, Ivan, did.

The wonderful thing is that this kind of complete healing is not reserved only for a handful of special students like Beth and Ivan. It is available to everyone. My vision is: a healer in every home and a world without pain and suffering. As Dr. Bill Manahan, a professor at the University of Minnesota Medical School, puts it, "Spring Forest Qigong is going to revolutionize the manner in which we look at healing."

Beth's story about healing breast cancer easily using the BodyMind is going to change how you look at healing, too.

Master Chunyi Lin
Author, *Born A Healer*
Spring Forest Qigong
www.springforestqigong.com
Eden Prairie, MN

FOREWORD

Beth Misner's eventful journey from the shock of a breast cancer diagnosis to vibrant health is incredibly inspiring, not just for those facing cancer or other life-threatening diseases, but for anyone aspiring to a higher level of vibrancy in their lives.

Ironically, Beth's breast cancer diagnosis came virtually on the heels of her and her husband, Ivan, releasing a book describing how he had healed from prostate cancer using natural methods. Beth's first reaction to hearing her small tumor was vascular and aggressive was laughter, as she realized she still had a lot to learn about healing. That positive start foreshadowed the relentlessly hopeful perspective she would bring to her future journey, to both the dark, shadowy valleys and the triumphant, sunlit peaks ahead.

In a dream Beth had immediately afterward, she dreamed that there was a hole under her house in which the inhabitants had been throwing their trash. The hidden pile caught alight and began to smolder, and her family waited nearby with a fire extinguisher until firemen arrived. Her two eldest children then discovered that the house had a previously unknown third floor attic. It was in a state of neglect.

Such symbolism is powerful and contains the seeds of understanding. Beth knew she had a competent medical support team, symbolized by the firefighters. Her children rallied around her and found the attic, a high dimension of Beth's psyche that, though neglected, was now identified and available to her.

Many cancer patients have warning dreams that are full of symbolism. A study by radiologist Larry Burk shows that the dreams have common characteristics: in

83 percent of cases, the dream is more intense and vivid than other dreams. Most dreamers experience a feeling of dread, and in 44 percent of cases, the word cancer or tumor appears.

In over half the cases Dr. Burk has collected, the dream resulted in the woman seeking medical consultation. Dreams led directly to diagnosis and frequently highlighted the precise location of the tumors.

As Beth took action and began to put together a treatment plan, she received a great deal of advice about both conventional and alternative treatments. Her balanced and well-informed approach to considering her options is a blueprint for any patient facing a life-threatening illness.

Beth and Ivan share with us in this book their celebration of successes and treatment milestones and the options they considered when there were difficult choices to be made along the path. They wisely include a common-sense section on what to do first, should you find yourself facing a cancer diagnosis.

Beth's story highlights the importance of getting informed about treatment choices and options, whatever medical challenges you are facing. It also reinforces the value of empowering the patient to make decisions.

Once Beth began to heal, she took a deeper look at her life. More than just wanting the cancer to go away, she wanted to find and discover what influences had triggered it in the first place. That would allow her to make changes that would eliminate behaviors and beliefs that were not serving her. Beth's focus on lifestyle change speaks to the fundamentals that underpin our health on a daily basis.

In the 1980s, I met a famous Russian healer named Victor Krivorotov. Victor's father had been a well-known healer, too, and people queued up around the block daily to receive his treatments.

Yet Victor eventually quit his practice because he observed that while energy healing produced apparent cures in most cases, patients invariably showed up later with relapses or new symptoms, because they had failed to change the beliefs and behaviors that contributed to their condition in the first place. Beth's first priority was eliminating every possible source of stress in her life. She then revised her schedule around a routine that supported a low-stress lifestyle.

It is difficult to overstate the impact of stress on disease. Research shows that adrenaline, one of our two primary stress hormones, promotes the metastasis of cancer and facilitates signaling between groups of cancer cells. Simultaneously, stress hormones act epigenetically to shut down genes that help our bodies identify and eliminate cancerous cells.

Not only is stress epigenetic, so is relaxation. When we meditate, become mindful, connect with nature, breathe consciously, use acupressure or acupuncture, or practice any one of the many forms of energy medicine, this signals our genes. In one study I did of a four-day meditation retreat, eight key genes were upregulated in participants, including three that play a role in suppressing tumors.

Beth came to realize that genes are like a deck of cards: it's not having a card in the deck that determines the game; it's which cards you play and how you play them that leads to a win. Our attitudes and behaviors are turning genes on and off moment by moment.

Part two of Beth's book covers advanced aspects of the Misner Plan, the method both Ivan and Beth used to heal their bodies. Co-authored with naturopath Betty Runkle, it includes a comprehensive review of the many natural healing methods available, along with the research that supports them. They range from fasting, Laetrile, and nutritional supplements to hyperbaric oxygen and a ketogenic diet. Some of these cancer treatments, while common in Europe and Asia, are unfortunately not available to US patients as cancer treatments. They may be accessed for building a stronger immune system, with the exception of Laetrile, which is still not permitted for use by doctors in our country.

The Misner Plan places a heavy emphasis on greatly reducing sugar from one's diet. This is essential, not just to remove the primary nutrient source for cancer cells, but also for overall health. Newer research is showing that even "healthy" sugars like the fructose found in fruit can be harmful in all but very small doses.

Beth also used energy methods like qigong and EFT (Tapping). A comprehensive bibliography maintained by the nonprofit that I chair, the National Institute for Integrative Healthcare (NIIH.org), contains over 600 studies showing the effectiveness of energy techniques for the following conditions:

Alzheimer's	HIV/AIDS
Anxiety	Insomnia
Arthritis	Irritable bowel syndrome
Asthma	Low back pain
Autism	Memory loss
Burnout	Menstrual distress
Burns	Migraines
Cancer	Mood disorders
Cardiovascular disease	Motion sickness
Carpal tunnel syndrome	Obesity
Children's behavioral issues	Pain
Cognitive impairment	Post-traumatic stress disorder
Cortisol excess	(PTSD)
Dementia	Prostate cancer
Depression	Pulmonary disease
Diabetes	Skin wounds
Drug addiction	Smoking
Fibromyalgia	Stroke
Headache	Substance abuse
High blood pressure	Thyroid dysfunction

While we can focus on the physical matter of our cells, molecules, and atoms, healing at the level of energy is elegant and effective.

Beth's story is like Beth herself—full of curiosity, joy, passion, goodwill, humor, and courage. You don't need to be facing cancer to benefit from the suggestions in these pages. The methods Beth and Ivan recommend produce a high-performance mind in a high-functioning body.

It is my sincere desire that Beth's extraordinary story inspires you to consider the possibilities for your life. Where are you stressing yourself and possibly triggering disease? What changes can you make to your thoughts and behaviors that will catalyze new levels of vibrancy? Knowing that we are affecting thousands of genes, hormones, and enzymes in our bodies, minds, and emotions empowers us all to make the most life-affirming choices.

Dawson Church
Author, *The Genie in Your Genes*

TABLE OF CONTENTS

PART ONE:
BETH'S JOURNEY

It's Time to Be Me
By Beth Misner

For many years, I've been many things.
Some of what I have been has served the goals of others.
Now I find myself in the second half of life,
And it's time to be me.

It's time to be the poet, the singer,
The artist, the author, the meditator.
It's time to set aside the to-do list
And time to start on the to-be list.
It's time to provide the cool refreshing oasis
To those in need of inspiration and peace.

When I'm true to myself,
What I have to offer is more meaningful.
When I'm walking in my gifts,
I can transmit the higher values.
When I'm being real, I'm doing well
And healing the body and the spirit.

The gift of cancer to my life
Can never be underestimated.
The messenger that came in the guise of a tumor
Whispered into my open heart:

"It's time to be you."

SETTING THE
STAGE TO HEAL

Beth

My gentle healing journey began with laughter. That was my spontaneous reaction to the results of my March 2017 breast-cancer screening by high-definition, color-Doppler ultrasound.

"This isn't good. You need to have this out," were the first words from my doctor when he saw the image on the ultrasound monitor.

He was looking at what appeared to be a 1.5 cm mass in my right breast with angiogenesis (blood flow), the hallmark of malignant tumors. He found a lymph node that looked "suspicious" that was also angiogenic.

But I'm getting ahead of myself.

My gentle healing journey actually started about one month earlier when I found a small, hard lump during my self-exam. I could tell this knot was not something like the frequent cysts I tend to get with hormonal cycles. It was firm and fixed: exactly what they tell you to be looking for when checking for breast cancer.

It had been my practice to use breast ultrasound yearly for my cancer screening after my first mammogram at age 40 (performed in 2004) came back with a suspicious result. I was referred at that time immediately to a breast-imaging center for the dreaded compression mammogram, in the days before 3D tomosynthesis mammograms existed. Fortunately, the compression mammo ruled out breast cancer, and the radiologist who performed the scan asked me if I would be interested in taking part in Dr. Kevin Kelly's clinical trial for his new automated breast ultrasound technology, SonoCine. Dr. Kelly was seeking to clinically prove that this new type of screening could detect smaller cancers sooner for women with dense breast tissue while resulting in higher accuracy due to the automated nature of the scan. It was truly a blessing to have been able to be part of this study.

Dr. Kelly was conducting studies at that time to seek FDA approval for automated breast ultrasound to be included in the early-screening procedures recommended by the American Medical Association and the American Cancer Society; he succeeded, and it was subsequently approved by the FDA for screening as an adjunct to mammography. Automated breast ultrasound has been detecting smaller malignant masses in women's breasts than mammograms can, and it does not expose the breast tissue to radiation, allowing for earlier intervention that is less damaging to overall health.

It had been my preferred method of breast-cancer screening from age 40 to 49, but after moving away from California in 2013, I had not found any radiology groups in Texas with the SonoCine automated breast ultrasound machine. So, I had started using thermography for my annual breast-cancer screening as I was under the impression that thermography would be a good, safe alternative.

I was in for a surprise.

The week following the self-exam where discovered the mass, I booked myself for a thermography scan. The technician who performed my thermography told me she could not (of course) reveal to me the results of the scan; I would have to wait for the doctors to review it and send me the report. What a tense wait that was. When I got the email in my inbox, I very eagerly opened the attached report and images. No detected angiogenesis. No cancer. All my lymph nodes were also cool. No angiogenesis. I was told, "Come back in a year."

Because there was some dimpling above the lump when the breast tissue was lifted, a friend of ours and contributing author, Dr. Mohammad Nikkhah, encouraged me not to stop there. "Go in for an ultrasound," he advised me. I'm so glad I listened to both him and my own intuition. I would later learn that older thermography cameras are only able to give the patient a certain amount of information. On my 2012 and 2013 scans, you can see some temperature variation right where the mass was, but since there was no change in the baseline thermography done in early 2012, the subsequent scans did not raise any alarms, although the tumor was already there and slowly becoming more invasive.

Dr. Kelly has baseline scans on me that go back twelve years. When I detected the lump, I consulted with him by phone, and then I flew to California from Texas to have him perform my high-definition, color Doppler ultrasound scan. Dr. Kelly had performed my husband, Ivan's, monthly ultrasound scans during the time his prostate cancer was reversing naturally as he followed specific alternative healthcare recommendations, so he was already well aware of the Misner Plan and also our particular mindset that our bodies can quickly heal themselves quite easily, even from cancer. If you've read *Healing Begins in the Kitchen*, you have already been introduced to Dr. Kelly.

So, there I was with Dr. Kelly, who explained to me what he was seeing in my breast tissue. When I saw Dr. Kelly's dour expression and then heard him say, "This isn't good. You need to have this out," I laughed because it seemed like some kind of cosmic joke. The exact word for the feeling in my heart in that moment was disbelief. I had been so certain that this lump was some kind of fibroid tumor: annoying but harmless.

When he turned on the color Doppler feature of the ultrasound, there was the evidence pointing to cancer: the orange, yellow, and white colors that indicate angiogenesis, the signature nature of increased blood flow within malignant tumors.

Benign tumors do not have capillaries feeding the cells within them. Cancer cells commandeer the body in such a way that they create capillaries to bring in

4

blood flow, so they can feed on sugars, iron, and other blood-borne nutrients. The edges of the mass were also jagged and uneven, in medical jargon–spiculated. It looked to me like one of Tim Burton's *Nightmare Before Christmas*–stylized trees.

Dr. Kelly took a closer look at the right axillary lymph node, pointing out to me that it had no white center, or hilum, and had more blood flow to it than would be normal. It was also quite enlarged and darker than the other, normal ones.

"This one is a problem, too," he told me.

Once again, just as with Ivan's prostate biopsy results appointment to which I had not gone, my husband and I were so confident that cancer was not one of the many possible outcomes for me that I had gone to my appointment in California without him. Thankfully, our eldest daughter, Ashley, who lives in the area, met me there and was with me for moral support.

But there I sat in Dr. Kelly's office, learning that cancer might also be part of my life, not just my husband's. I had some very conflicting feelings about that possibility. I mean, we were just about to release our first book about healing cancer naturally, and I was learning that I was on the verge of a metastatic breast cancer diagnosis! How ironic. And how was it that I could have a cancer diagnosis looming when I had been following the Misner Plan for the previous five years? What did this mean for the efficacy of our plan? We would learn later that I had gene mutations that played into this situation, but I did not know about that until sometime later.

After I laughed, my next thought to myself was, *well, it looks like I have more to learn about healing cancer naturally!*

I had made arrangements to travel back to Austin immediately after my appointment with Dr. Kelly. I sat on the plane shell-shocked, a million thoughts running through my head, but I can honestly tell you not one second was spent experiencing any fear.

In our first book, *Healing Begins in the Kitchen*, about Ivan's prostate cancer diagnosis and subsequent remission after changing his diet, we wrote about how my mother chose alternative healthcare after her cancer diagnosis when I was a child. She eventually did have surgery to remove a tumor in her colon. Her tumor had already begun to shrink from the natural therapies she pursued. I was raised with an understanding that chemotherapy, surgery, and radiation are not the only ways to approach a cancer diagnosis. I believe that the "standard of care" in the United States is often not the most effective way to heal cancer. And I had heard about others, not only Ivan, who completely reversed their cancers (often in the very late stages, too) and went on to live long, healthy lives.

No, I was not afraid.

Dr. Kelly had told me that this lump was small enough that a competent surgeon could remove it easily, possibly with a simple lumpectomy. "Get a good breast guy right away," he told me. I came back to Austin to consider what to do next. We have a BNI member in Austin, Tom Schnorr, who studied at the University of Texas Health Science Center for his Ph.D. in pharmacology. I went straight into his compounding pharmacy to ask him for a good referral to a surgeon. Without hesitation, he said, "MD Anderson in Houston. Don't go anywhere else." So, I made that call. Beth Misner, the co-author of *Healing Begins in the Kitchen,* called MD Anderson for a surgical consultation with an oncologist.

I'll never forget the email that quickly came in from my mom after she learned about my decision. She had a very bad feeling about me going to a conventional "cancer doctor." She was concerned I would become scared, and then I might step onto a path that would pull me deeper into the "standard of care" mindset and lead me to complications and further degradation of my health and my life. She felt certain the MD Anderson doctor would likely intimidate me with the intensity of conviction that I needed to move fast and that chemotherapy and surgery with possible radiation afterwards would be the only things she would place any hope in for my survival if my tumor and lymph node were indeed malignant.

I reassured Mom that I wanted to access all the tools available to me, and MD Anderson would have the very best diagnostic tests available. If a lumpectomy

BETH MISNER

were possible, it could likely be done there with alacrity and ease. I'm not sure she believed me completely, but she seemed to feel better after hearing my thoughts.

My mom has been my first source of inspiration to pursue natural healing, and my husband has been my second. Both of their experiences have opened my eyes to the possibility of shrinking tumors naturally and even resolving them completely.

Since my appointment with the oncologist was two weeks down the road, I used that time to begin my alternative healthcare in Austin, approaching it as if I already had confirmation that the mass was malignant. My rationale: Dr. Kelly has seen enough malignant masses in his many, many years in practice that when he feels as confident as he did with me that this was cancer, there was a strong likelihood he was correct. I also realized that if my body had developed a tumor, even if it was not malignant, there was a problem in my immune system somewhere, and I wanted to support my body in healing any kind of tumor–malignant or benign.

I started having hyperbaric chamber sessions three times per week, and my integrative medicine physician's assistant at the Westlake Medical Arts Center ordered vitamin C and glutathione IVs for me in order to support my immune function. She also ordered a battery of blood tests that showed I had very high inflammatory markers (both sedimentation rate and C-reactive protein), and my white blood cell count was quite low, indicating that my immune system was not functioning well. It did not behave as if it were aware that there was anything wrong in my body. She encouraged me to step out of my volunteer role with the BNI Foundation and take a total "time out" in order to allow myself to rest and de-stress.

"You have enough on your plate right now with this new development," she wisely counseled. She also recommended that I look into low-dose Naltrexone, a drug usually given in high doses to help people get off opiates or alcohol dependence. In low doses, it has been shown to increase the body's production of serotonin, boosting one's immune function.

Taking her advice, I also turned my cell phone's notifications off—Facebook, Twitter, Instagram, Pinterest, What'sApp, news feeds—and I completely eliminated my work schedule—business calls and video meetings with quite a few groups of folks that had been filling up my days. I told everyone I was putting myself in what I lovingly came to see as a personal friend: my Healing Bubble. I plugged into quiet, contemplative meditation, morning t'ai chi and qigong practice, journaling and prayer, as well as simply sitting by my pool reading magazines. I started re-learning how to breathe deeply, realizing that I had spent a large part of each day either breathing shallowly or actually holding my breath for long stretches of time.

The other thing I did was to recommit to following the dietary protocol of our Misner Plan. Prior to this, I had been relaxing my discipline on what I would allow myself to eat or drink, and I was putting non-Misner Plan foods in my body fairly regularly. In the interest of full disclosure, I will share with you that I had started slipping the occasional peppermint pattie in with the groceries and ordering a freshly baked apple fritter at the local farmer's market on occasion. I actually said out loud once or twice: "I don't have cancer. I can eat that . . ."

It suddenly dawned on me that the whole time I was saying, thinking, and doing those things, I may have been feeding cancer cells, because cancer loves sugar. Ivan encouraged me not to beat myself up over it. It is what it is, and we have dealt with it with all the resources to which we had access. I have realized that one never really knows for sure, so for me, I became much more motivated at that time to eat "as if" I didn't want to feed cancer cells.

I'm reminded of the wise words of our good friend, Stewart Emery, about the need to have a heart-centered approach to food: "It is one thing to eat foods for the nourishment of our bodies and another still to be afraid of certain foods, or to demonize an entire food group." I want what I eat to fill my senses, to bring me pleasure, and to unlock my body's healing potential. I don't want to live in fear of certain foods.

For more details on my diet and our approach to nutrition and cancer, please read *Healing Begins in the Kitchen: Get Well and Stay There on the Misner Plan.* The focus of this book will not be on the dietary approach of the Misner Plan.

I had a dream during this time frame that I knew was meaningful the instant I woke up. I dreamt that I was in my house, and there was a hole in the floor into which we put all our trash. Underneath the floor was a flow of water that carried the trash out of our home. The cover over this hole had slipped off and revealed smoke from a fire smoldering somewhere below the floor. I knew instantly where the fire extinguisher was, but I could not put out the fire, because I couldn't see its source. I called 911, reported the fire, and took comfort from the assurance of knowing that the professionals were on the way. I relaxed, confident that they would know how to manage the fire.

While I waited in the dream for the firefighters to arrive on the scene, my two eldest children called for me to come upstairs with them. They had found something to show me. My son, Trey, stayed by the hole in the floor with the extinguisher, in case the flames started coming up into the house, and I followed my other two children, Ashley and Dorian, to see what it was they had found.

"There's a whole third floor to our house up here, Mom," they told me.

"What?" I exclaimed. "How did I not know that?"

As we went up a flight of stairs to a finished attic on the third floor, I noticed it was all dusty and dirty, and the furniture up there was covered with sheets and plastic. All around on the walls were murals of cathedrals and churches from England and France. It was lovely. And very much in a state of neglect. I knew I needed to dust everything off, open up the windows, and begin using this part of my house.

Later when I woke up, I wrote this dream down and let its message come into my heart. I had known that I had something going on in my body. Five years prior to this time, before I moved to Austin, Dr. Bill Kellas of the Center for Advanced Medicine in Encinitas, California, had told me that there was something smoldering somewhere in my body. I had a blood test that came back with an extremely high C-reactive protein level, one of the markers of inflammation. We did a lot of other testing, but nothing specific showed up. He literally said the words, "Beth, there is a fire simmering somewhere."

In the dream, I knew I had a remedy at hand, and I also knew I needed to call in professionals to help. But there was no sense of fear in the dream that the fire was going to become so big that the house would be destroyed. I took comfort from this message my spirit was sending me.

The professionals were on the way. I was going to be fine.

I interpreted the dream to also be redirecting me to the part of my life that had been devoted to spiritual development and growth. I could see how I had neglected this aspect of my life for a few years, and I knew it was time to open the figurative windows, let light in, and dust off the cobwebs that had formed.

This dream became even more significant to me once I studied how our subconscious minds communicate with both our conscious minds and our bodies.

As long as I live, I'll never forget the appointment at MD Anderson with the oncologist, a breast surgeon. Even before I went in for the appointment, I could tell I was plugging into a huge machine. I began to receive emails with links to the incredibly well-designed and informative patient portal. I had a long call with a patient navigator. I had never even heard of a patient navigator before. When Ivan and I arrived at the office after a three-hour drive from Austin to the Houston area, I was checked in and given my patient ID number and a spiffy wristband. I started to feel a little bit of tingling sensation around the edges of my brain. I wouldn't say it was fear, but it was definitely discomfort.

When Ivan and I went in to see the surgeon, she listened to my experience up to that point, reviewed Dr. Kelly's report, examined both of my breasts, nodded, and got out her black Sharpie marker. She put two X marks on my right breast, one where the lump could be felt and one on the opposite side of my breast, directly across from the lump. This was getting more and more real.

Then she told me what she wanted to do right there on the spot: "I want to send you over to our radiology department. They are standing by, waiting for you right now. I want you to have a mammogram, another ultrasound, and a biopsy today, so I can advise you on how we are going to proceed."

Cue the scratching sound on the vinyl record.

Biopsy? I was, and still am, completely opposed to having a biopsy. No oncologist or surgeon can (or will) tell you that there is zero risk of releasing circulating tumor cells when performing a biopsy. Called "tracking," there is, in fact, a certain amount of risk with biopsies that cells which can seed new tumors may be released from the primary tumor if it is malignant. I knew this from the research Ivan and I had done together when he was healing prostate cancer naturally. My gut instinct also questioned the idea of puncturing a suspected malignant tumor and allowing that tumor to bleed into the healthy tissue. It seemed to me that would further inflame an already inflammatory condition and might also allow tumor cells to be carried into my blood stream or lymphatic system. That was not something I wanted to allow to happen.

When I asked her if the information she would gain from the biopsy would change the treatment plan, her response was: "The standard of care is to perform the biopsy, then I will have the information I need to determine what kind of chemotherapy to use first to shrink the tumor before we even consider any surgical procedure. Without a biopsy, I cannot even recommend a treatment plan, so there is no way for me to answer that question."

Perplexed about how to proceed, I looked at Ivan with a lost expression on my face. He looked back at me reassuringly, and I knew from the expression in his eyes that he would support whatever decision I made in the moment. It was one of those unspoken exchanges of clear communication between two people who know each other well. Even so, I think I surprised him when I acquiesced and got the information about where to go for the diagnostic tests. Once we were out in the car, I was able to share with him what my thought process was: I wanted more information. I needed more information. An ultrasound cannot give the whole picture with breast cancer. And I knew that the radiologist would be the one to perform the ultrasound-guided biopsy she felt was indicated after doing the scans. If the radiologist could perform an excisional biopsy, she might remove the lump altogether if it were small enough for that to be possible. In that case, I would not need to depend on the oncologist to stage the cancer in order to have the lump removed. I was not considering how I would approach the lymph node in question.

I told him, "I can always refuse the biopsy if the information from the scans indicates that there is something more than this tiny lump."

I knew I was not there to consider receiving the traditional standard of care.

On the short drive to the radiology center, we called Dr. Mohammad, who had been so helpful with Ivan's cancer-healing process. He agreed that the information we were going to gain from the diagnostic tests would help me in making my next decision. And he encouraged me to consider allowing a biopsy if it looked like surgery could be done in the next two weeks. This would minimize the risk of the tumor "growing" from the needle aspiration. He also confirmed my presumption that I could refuse the biopsy when it got to that point if it looked like the situation were more complicated or that there was more there than we already knew about.

You see, I had already decided when I was a young pre-teen that the medical standard of care would not be the only thing, or even the first thing, I would consider if I were to be diagnosed with cancer. I had even told Ivan before we were married: "If I am ever diagnosed with something like breast cancer, I plan to go to Mexico for a month and come home healed." My decision had already been made. But in this situation, I needed more information to know if I was going to act on that decision or not. I was open to having an excisional biopsy as a starting point to completely remove the tumor, if that were possible, before doubling down on other alternative healthcare options to correct the root cause for my body's creation of a tumor, malignant or not.

THE GAME IS AFOOT

Beth

When we arrived at the radiology center, we both noticed something very strange in the waiting room. There was a large floor banner with the MD Anderson logo and their tag line. The way the banner was laid out graphically, the message they were conveying was probably not the one they wanted to get across. At the top of the banner was the word CANCER written in uppercase letters in white. The word was crossed out in red and the words Be Afraid were written in red beside it.

All I could see was, "Be Afraid" like a bright red warning light flashing on and off. I am not afraid of cancer, but this sign heightened my fear of the standard of care, which has been proved to be carcinogenic in and of itself. Chemotherapy is known to be carcinogenic. Radiation is known to be carcinogenic. Cancer can spread in the body as a result of biopsies and repeat biopsies. I sat there in that waiting room intentionally focusing on all I know about how the body can powerfully heal when supported adequately in order to relax my BodyMind and keep fear from coming into my experience.

When I was called back to begin the diagnostic procedure, I knew each step I was taking was literally carrying me closer to the path I needed to be on to heal. I kept saying to myself, "I need the information." Ivan was allowed to wait in a private waiting room while I was having the diagnostic tests.

The 3D mammogram (digital breast tomosynthesis) was intense. My breasts

14

became so painful from the amount of pressure used to flatten my sensitive tissue that I could not even wear my seatbelt across my chest for weeks! And flattening the tissue in the armpit area? Forget about it! I would not have thought what they were able to do was even physically possible. I felt like someone had just punched on me under my arm. And I wondered how much more inflammation was created by this kind of rough treatment of my breasts and lymph nodes, not to mention the barrage of x-rays to this area. I am a black belt in karate; I know how to take the punches, and this was intensely painful with the pain lasting a good two weeks later.

After performing the mammogram, the technician asked me if I would be willing to consider a core biopsy. That encouraged me because I thought that perhaps she had been able to tell that the mass was small enough to simply biopsy it out. Before being called in for the ultrasound, I was able to share that tidbit with Ivan in the waiting room. We both felt very relieved.

I went into the ultrasound scan with a much lighter heart. The technician did a very thorough scan, but the pressure she used only added to the painfulness of my breast tissue. After the scan, the technician excused herself to review the findings with the radiologist.

Dr. Monica Huang came to my side about five minutes later. She gently laid her hand on my right forearm and said, "Well, there is a lot more going on than just the lump you can feel."

I took a deep breath in and slowly released it.

"Tell me," I quietly responded with peace in my heart, ready to receive the information I needed in order to be able to make the decision about what I was going to do.

She continued, "In addition to the primary mass, which is about 3 centimeters in diameter, there are two suspicious calcifications that are metabolically active. This brings the total dimension of the area of suspicion to 5 centimeters, and there is also the one involved axillary node. I want to do a core biopsy of the main

15

mass, two needle biopsies of the calcifications, and a needle biopsy of the lymph node."

I put my left hand over her hand, which was still resting on my arm.

I calmly said, "I am going to decline the biopsies. This is not my path. I plan to use alternative care to heal."

Her response was great.

She told me, "I completely respect your decision, and I'm here for anything else you may need. Just call me. Anytime." She gave me her business card with her direct line on it.

I got up off the examination table, returned to the locker room to dress, and then went into the private waiting room where Ivan was sitting. He could tell immediately from my expression that the news had not been what we had been hoping for.

"There's more than just the one mass. There isn't going to be any core biopsy or needle biopsies. There is too much in there for a lumpectomy," I told him as I drew in another long, deep breath.

It was then that I felt myself going into a panic attack. That had happened to me not long before this experience when a flight we were on had trouble landing in bad weather in Central Texas. After circling the Austin airfield and trying three times to land in thick clouds with intense turbulence, we were diverted to land in San Antonio. While flying to San Antonio, we learned that the plane was running low on fuel. It was a very tense 45-minute incident. Once we had landed, my entire body began to shake uncontrollably. I was mentally calm, but the adrenaline that my body released during the incident put me into a state of psychological shock. The same thing started to happen in the waiting room. I felt like I was having an out-of-body experience. Once again, I was calm in my heart and my mind, but my body was reacting to the adrenaline released in my body after hearing the words: "There is a lot more going on than just the lump."

"I need to get out of here," I told my husband as I started trembling.

We gathered all our things and headed straight out to the car. Later I would reflect that I should have asked to look at the scans with Dr. Huang, so I could have understood more about what she was seeing. I should have asked questions, but instead, I felt like I needed to just get as far away from MD Anderson as I could.

We quickly got on the road home to Austin. My husband is my biggest supporter. He has never wavered in his attitude that I need to make my own decisions, even if they are different from his own ideas and preferences. He had said, with regard to his own experience in healing cancer naturally, that he needed to be the captain of his own ship, and he was now extending that grace to me.

"You need to do what you feel is best, honey," he told me in the car as we drove home.

I wanted to consult with a couple of the doctors who had been working with him at Clínica CIPAG in Tijuana, Mexico, before making my decision regarding what direction to go in next. Ivan told me that I had his complete support and freedom to go in the direction I felt was best for me.

Although prostate cancer and breast cancer are related in that they are both considered to be reproductive cancers and are usually influenced by hormones, there are significant differences. Dr. Mohammad shared with me subsequently that it could be easier to heal breast cancer naturally than prostate cancer. I felt particularly encouraged by that since Ivan had healed prostate cancer once using natural therapies and integrative medicine and probably again when it looked like he had come out of remission. I also realized that, whereas he had only developed cancer in one place, it looked like I possibly already had metastatic disease.

Nevertheless, Ivan's profound healing experience gave me the confidence to stay positive and focused throughout my own healing process. He was, and still is, my rock.

My appointment at MD Anderson had taken place on Friday. I took the weekend to talk to my practitioners, research breast cancer diagnosis procedures, and come up with my next steps. It was important to me to get the information I needed and make my own decision. I did not want to be told one way was the *only* way to approach recovering my health. I learned over the weekend that a large percentage of women who have a positive mammogram and ultrasound later learn through biopsy that their tumors are benign. I also learned even more about the effect of tracking and seeding new tumors through biopsy. It was, more than ever, not something I wanted to have done to me.

I wondered if a 3T (three Tesla magnets instead of two—giving a clearer image) MRI, the same diagnostic test Ivan had been having to track the progression of his prostate cancer healing, would be a less invasive confirmation of Dr. Huang's suspicions. On Monday, I took her up on her offer to call her anytime.

"Yes, that sounds like a reasonable direction to go. I'd be happy to perform your scan, if you'd like me to," she reassured me when I asked her about the scan. Not wanting to have another long drive ahead of us, I told her I would ask my local practitioner to order the scan. She agreed with that and asked me to keep her updated.

My 3T MRI was scheduled for Wednesday. With all breast cancer scans, a Bi-Rads score should be reported to gauge the likelihood that a suspicious spot is malignant or not; sometimes you have to ask your doctor what your score is, because they do not automatically share that with the patient. The higher the score, the more likely it is that the suspicious lesion is malignant. A Bi-Rads 6 score is given to a lesion that has been confirmed by a tissue biopsy to be malignant. Both of my previous ultrasounds and mammogram had returned with a Bi-Rads 5 score, which indicated "highly likely for malignancy." I talked it over with Ivan, and we agreed that if my 3T MRI came back with a Bi-Rads 5 score, I would begin alternative treatment in Mexico right away. I was not going to do a

18

biopsy. I did not want to take the risk of spreading more circulating tumor cells than were possibly already shed by a malignant tumor into my bloodstream. I was okay proceeding as if I had the confirmation that the tumor, the calcifications, and the suspicious lymph gland were malignant.

Some people would not have been content to approach their situation this way. I have had interactions and experiences with other women who have felt they needed absolute confirmation before taking the steps I took. I have also known women for whom it was their spouses who were the ones who felt they needed to have cellular confirmation, meaning a tissue biopsy. Unwilling to take the risk of seeding new tumors through tracking, we studied the reliability of other types of lab tests to give us confirmation of cancer. I will be sharing what these tests are as my story unfolds.

I started looking into clinics in Mexico. I emailed Dr. Castillo at Clínica CIPAG, where Ivan had gone twice for treatment for prostate cancer, and then I waited for his response. In the meantime, I got online and researched the non-toxic immunotherapy done at the Issels ImmunoOncology Hospital in Tijuana, Mexico, with follow-up care to build up my own immune function at the Issels Medical Center in Santa Barbara, CA. Their approach is similar to Clínica CIPAG's, but they also create cancer vaccines out of the patient's own immune cells to wake up the immune system in order to heal cancer. They specialize in late-stage cancer, so I felt that my very early, possibly stage 2 status would respond well to this approach. I also liked the idea of being in Mexico for one week and then continuing treatment in California for three weeks in order to bring my immune system fully online.

While I was waiting to go in for my 3T MRI in order to evaluate the cellular differentiation (poor cellular differentiation would be a more conclusive sign that the tumor was malignant), I completed the intake forms for the Issels' treatment program and submitted the application along with copies of my diagnostic reports to find out if they would accept me into their treatment program.

Two days later, I went in for the 3T MRI. As is the normal practice, the technician performing the scan gave me absolutely no indication if there was poor cell differentiation within the tumor and the lymph node. It was frustrating to know she knew—she was standing right in front of me with that knowledge—and I still had to wait for the report to be sent to my doctor!

The waiting game commenced.

While I was waiting for the results of the scan, I was accepted into the Issels' natural immune therapy program on Friday. I booked my flight from Austin to San Diego for two days later, Sunday, to be admitted into Hospital Los Angeles in Tijuana, Mexico. Dr. Castillo emailed me just before I departed for Mexico.

"You're in good hands," he told me upon reading my decision to enter the Issels Immune Therapy program.

WINGMAN FOR MY WIFE

Ivan

I was concerned when Beth found the small lump in her breast, and at the same time, I was not extremely worried. She had had cysts before, and initially, I tried to be as reassuring as I could be that this was most likely another cyst. But as time went on, there was no doubt that this mass was distinctly different.

I tried to be positive for her, encouraging her to do what she needed to do in order to decide where to go for treatment if she ended up needing to do that. It was important to me that I let her know she was in the pilot's seat with me at her side as her wingman. Her attitude was positive from the very beginning. There was only one day through this entire healing journey when she really struggled to stay positive, which let me know that this was weighing heavily on her mind, even though she was upbeat and so strong.

I thought I had been positive when facing my own healing from cancer. But Beth put me to shame. She was the epitome of positivity, centeredness, and courage that one needs when healing cancer naturally.

Another conflict I had was that she kept insisting that I stick to our travel plans to visit our BNI markets in South Korea and India. We had planned a two-week trip together, and she now felt she should go straight into treatment. I was completely willing to cancel my trips so I could travel with her to Mexico and then to Santa Barbara, but she felt strongly that I needed to stick to the plans to visit our BNI members in the two countries while she was admitted into the hospital.

"The members have already planned to see you, the regions have booked venues, and contracts for the events have been signed," she said. "I will be fine there, and I'm not having any surgeries or other invasive procedures. We've been to Mexico twice before for your treatment. I'm comfortable going on my own, and I speak Spanish," she rationally insisted.

I had such mixed emotions, but I also felt the same way she did about the commitments made by the franchise owners in our international regions to have me come in to speak for their members.

The fact that she was not feeling ill at all but rather was feeling strong, upbeat, and completely healthy made it a little bit easier for me to accept her decision to go straight to Mexico. I was completely torn but accepted her decision and request that I travel while she was in treatment.

During the time I was overseas, we had regular contact through emails and phone calls. I'll let her share more about her experiences, but it was clear to me that she was thriving under the treatments and that she was feeling great about her choice to follow the Issels protocol. That really allowed me to relax and be present for the BNI events, although she was constantly on my mind and in my heart, as you might imagine.

At every event I attended, our BNI members asked me over and over how she was doing and told me to let her know they were thinking of her, praying for her, and sending love. I know this was very encouraging for her, too. They showered me with gifts to bring back to her—so many gifts that I had to have boxes shipped home because I could not carry them all back in my luggage! I got incense, healing beads, oils, mushroom extracts—you name it.

After Beth's hospitalization in Mexico and three weeks' treatment in Santa Barbara, I flew to California to be with her for the last few days and to travel down to Pasadena for her one-month scan to see how the Issels protocol had impacted the tumor and lymph gland. It was such a relief for us both to be together again. And I am so proud of how hard she worked and how positive she stayed. Every time I had called her from the road, I heard in her voice how well she was doing.

I had taken healing naturally from prostate cancer seriously, really focusing on all the things I needed to do to regain my health. And Beth took it all much further than I did. Where I had taken a look at the Good, Better, Best approaches and picked mostly from the Best column for the Misner Plan, Beth chose only from the Best column. I'm convinced that is part of the reason why her recovery was so rapid.

I had done body-mind techniques during my healing process, including regular meditation and some qigong exercises. I worked to greatly reduce the stressors in my life, which are known to suppress one's immune system. But most of my focus was on dietary changes. I slowly and steadily healed completely the first time, and when it looked like I may have come out of remission, I refocused on my dietary strategy and included the healing therapies being done at Clínica CIPAG. You can read more about my treatment in *Healing Begins in the Kitchen*. My body recovered quickly the second time around but not nearly as fast as Beth's body responded to all the body-mind techniques that she made a daily part of her healing journey. She also included electrical cellular treatments and quantum biofeedback, which I did not do.

But I'll let her tell you more about her treatment.

OFF TO MEXICO

Beth

The fact that I had made the decision to choose alternative healthcare for cancer when I was so young (and announced it to my soon-to-be husband at the age of 24, as I have already mentioned) made implementing my choice easy. I had already seen Ivan heal, so I was confident that I could also experience healing, even though I had a lymph node involved in an apparent metastasis. And I was not completely sure yet whether or not the Bi-Rads 5 scores could be explained some other way, such as a type of fungi, known as sac fungi, which mimics cancer in scans.

We went to the airport together, Ivan bound for South Korea and me for San Diego. It was a bittersweet parting at the gate when my flight boarded. I was going to miss my husband dearly, but I felt like we had made the right decision. I would later understand that it was important for my psyche that I took myself down there immediately—and that I went alone. I had a lot to prove to myself over the next four weeks.

I was met at the San Diego airport by the hospital's driver, who took me straight across the border to Hospital Los Angeles in a 25-minute drive. The admission procedure was smooth and quick. I got settled into my little room. This room was to become like a mountaintop cave in which I would nourish both my soul and my body for the next week.

Once I was settled in my room, I met with one of my doctors, Dr. Hector

Torres. He explained what was going to transpire over the next week and answered my questions. He told me that I would be seeing my other two treating physicians daily and that he would be seeing me twice per day. We hit it off very well, and he was interested in my mental focus: the qigong and meditation with which I was going to supplement my treatment.

When he got ready to leave, he asked me if I wanted some lunch. I had arrived after lunchtime, and I knew that the kitchen was done serving. Not wanting to trouble them, I told him, "No, I'm okay." But in reality, I was very hungry! It was in that instant that I realized I should be asking for what I knew I needed. I would later analyze why that was so hard for me, realizing it might be part of why I found myself in this situation. I quickly changed my answer, letting him know that I was hungry and would very much appreciate having something to eat. A delicious, natural protein shake was sent up to my room.

Before going into the hospital, I had told my friends and posted on Facebook that I was going to be staying off social media during my treatment in order to stay focused on healing. I was creating a Healing Bubble so I had the space and energy to be single-minded in my healing. I did, however, start a private, closed group on Facebook where I could post something daily and request support, prayer, encouragement, and at times humor, to support my process. I also requested and received a full medical leave from my role as co-founder of the BNI Foundation, as well as secretary of the foundation's board.

Day one, Monday, dawned brightly. The meals being served by the hospital were very congruent with the Misner Plan. The Issels Hospital believes in making sure patients have something to eat every two to three hours, so I was served three meals and three snacks each day. And the food was fresh, organic, and either steamed or served raw. I received a binder with the Issels protocol spelled out and lots of recipes for the patients to use when they returned home.

After my breakfast, Dr. Torres and a nurse came in. Dr. Torres explained what was going to happen during my first full day in the hospital, and then I had blood drawn in quite a number of vials for them to test all my lab values. I also received my IV catheter, which would remain in place during my stay, and my first multi-vitamin, multi-mineral IV infusion.

While I was receiving the infusion, my 3T MRI report arrived in my email from my doctor in Austin. This scan also came back with a Bi-Rads 5 score: highly suspicious for malignancy. I forwarded this report to Dr. Kelly, and I requested a phone consultation with him.

Later that day when my infusion was finished, I was looking for a way to exercise, so I ran the stairs of the six-story hospital. The nurses at the nurses' station looked at me with disbelief when I came down the hall dressed in workout clothes and told them what I was going to do. It felt so good to get my blood flowing and to breathe deeply. I came back to my room and did crunches and push-ups, and then I spent the rest of the day learning more about cancer vaccines, the immune system, and the Issels protocol.

Before supper, my three doctors came in to see how I was doing. They shared that they would be able to give me a report later during the week to let me know how many circulating tumor (cancer) cells (CTCs), if any, were in the blood they were going to collect to make my vaccines and how many immune cells were also present. I was very anxious to get that pathology report. It would confirm the status of the tumor without a biopsy. It would also have a count of the additional cancer cells circulating in my bloodstream that cannot seed new tumors so are not considered tumor cells. This count would also give them an idea of the severity of my condition. They would also be able to use the CTC and other "daughter" cells to phenotype my particular cancer. That would let them know if I had an aggressive type of cancer or one of the more indolent mutations.

I was able to talk to Ivan in Seoul, South Korea, before going to sleep that night, which was just wonderful. He was so encouraging and completely supportive. I fell asleep with a smile on my face.

The next morning, I got up, had a time of meditation, and did a short qigong practice. After that, all three of my treating doctors paid me a short visit in order to let me know what to expect from day two. I was going to be giving about a pint of blood so they could make the vaccines for me out of my immune cells, and then I would be getting a Laetrile (vitamin B_{17}) infusion, after which I could rest, read, and watch TV, if I wanted to. Laetrile is considered non-toxic chemotherapy. Laetrile is selective in weakening cancer cells only but was banned as a cancer treatment by the FDA in the United States after a lot of controversy. Ivan had also received Laetrile infusions while being treated at Clínica CIPAG. And my mother had received Laetrile in the early 70s when she was treated at an alternative healthcare clinic in Colorado.

Dr. Torres came in again to get me ready to have my immune cells harvested. He showed me a slide show that explained what they were going to do and gave me a chance to ask the million questions I had.

"I'm ready," I finally told him after he patiently answered all my questions.

"Great," he responded. "Let's get started."

The nurse came in with her supplies and drew the blood from which my immature immune cells (lymphocytes) and dendritic cells would be extracted so they could be treated in the lab to become activated and powerful.

As the bag began to fill with my blood, I began to sense the life pulsating in that bag—my life! I held the bag for a moment before the nurse took it off to the lab to do their magic, and I talked to my cells, telling them to train hard, that I loved them and could not wait for them to get back into my body. I was sure the nurse thought I was crazy, but Dr. Torres seemed to be particularly supportive of my desire to hold my cells and make sure they knew I loved them.

After Dr. Torres left to take my blood to the lab, the nurse started the Laetrile infusion. I began listening to the Audible book I downloaded before arriving: *Love, Medicine, and Miracles* by Dr. Bernie Siegel. Dr. Siegel wrote about what he calls exceptional patients, sharing from his years of experience with cancer patients which ones he saw healed more thoroughly and quickly. These exceptional patients kept their attitudes positive and hopeful. They were involved in the decisions about their care. They asked questions, read additional materials about their conditions and their treatment, and had other practices that kept them focused and calm, such as prayer and meditation.

I had read this book a couple of times in the months after Ivan's first achievement of remission from cancer. Now that I was the one in the healing mode, I wanted to digest Dr. Siegel's content with my own situation in mind. I intended to be one of those exceptional patients.

Later on that day, I was able to have another call with Dr. Mohammad. He gave me additional healing prescriptions: spend at least an hour each day doing two things that would lift my spirit. He told me to watch funny YouTube videos and laugh until I'd cry. He also said to read or watch very heart-warming stories such as the ones in Jack Canfield's *Chicken Soup for the Soul* series. He explained that these two prescriptions would cue my brain to release hormones that would strengthen my immune system. I took his advice to heart and have done this daily now since that time. I think I laughed that first night more than I had laughed in at least six months. It felt so good to release deep belly laughter until tears rolled down my cheeks.

I got into a routine of getting up, meditating, and doing my qigong practice, and having breakfast. Then I got myself all set up in the recliner next to my bed with my journal, books, iPad, and music before the nurse came in to start my infusions—multi-vitamins, multi-minerals, and Laetrile. I also was given oxygen treatments to be sure my blood oxygen saturation rate was very high.

One of many good things I have to say for the Issels ImmunoOncology Hospital is that they certainly do feed the patients well. In addition to meals and snacks, I was able to order protein drinks or fresh juices if I needed more nourishment. Every time the orderly arrived with food, I sent up a cheer. It was good to get the great food and equally nice to see someone to share a smile and a friendly word with.

On my third day in the hospital, I was able to talk with Dr. Kelly so he could explain the results of my 3T MRI in layman's terms. He told me the cell differentiation in both the tumor and the lymph node was not good, which is typical of malignancies. He also was able to anticipate from the results that I would not be dealing with intraductal carcinoma, but rather intralobular carcinoma. Although spread out more widely than intraductal cancer, intralobular cancer typically has fewer cancer cells contained in the affected area. He stressed again that I needed to do something quickly because it had become invasive at this point and had apparently metastasized. This was not a case of "in situ" any longer.

It felt good to be able to tell him that I was actually on day 3 of my treatment, and I made an appointment for a follow-up scan with him immediately after concluding the Issels program and before going home to Austin.

RECEIVING THE VACCINES

Beth

On Wednesday, Dr. Torres sat with me for quite a long time to explain what would be happening on days four and five. I was all set to receive the first half of my own activated T-cells into my body through an IV infusion on Thursday. Called autologous lymphokine-activated killer (LAK) cells, these lymphocytes are matured and multiplied in the lab. They are then activated to break down cancer cells in the presence of Interleuken-2 (a specific protein used by immune cells to signal for support when cancer cells are encountered). The autologous natural killer (NK) cells are also lymphocytes of the innate immune system that are matured and multiplied in the presence of Interleuken-21 and special cytokines (proteins) and activated to destroy cancer cells.

He explained that if everything went as expected, I might begin to feel sick right away, which would be good. Since these cells were being matured in the lab and activated to make them aggressive in my body against cancer cells, they would most likely trigger a rather intense immune response from the rest of my immune system. I could expect to get a sore throat, feel flu-like symptoms, or even run a fever.

We also talked about whether or not I wanted to receive an intra-tumoral injection with a small syringe of the autologous LAK/NK cells. I asked a *ton* of questions, specifically about what the risks would be of spreading cancer by injecting this tumor. Dr. Torres shared with me that the optimal time to do the intra-tumoral injection would be on Friday, after I had already had the LK/NAK infusion and the activated dendritic cells. My whole immune system would be on high alert, so if any more circulating tumor cells were released, they would be quickly neutralized.

I asked him to let me think about it, talk to a couple of people, do some research, and let him know in the morning. He agreed with that plan of action.

He then went on to explain that on Friday I would be receiving an injection of my own (autologous) dendritic cells that had been isolated at the same time as the circulating tumor cells and all the malignant daughter cells contained in the blood I had given. The second half of the autologous dendritic cells would be frozen and sent home with me to be injected subcutaneously in two weeks' time. I decided to call them the pit bulls because I thought of them as my guards.

Here is a description of the autologous dendritic cell vaccine from the Issels' website: "Dendritic cells are key regulators of immune responses and orchestrate innate and adaptive immunities. They are the most potent antigen-presenting cells and have the potential to invoke an anti-tumor immune response. The vaccine is cultured from the patient's own peripheral monocytes in the presence of a recombinant growth factor, special cytokines, and the patient's own tumor antigens, which are fractionated into peptides in order to achieve a more specific immune response."

Autologous cytokines, or Interleuken-2, (IL-2) were being prepared for me to take with me so I could give myself an injection of them every two weeks for six months. IL-2 would continue stimulating the new immune cells, or lymphocytes, my body would be producing on an ongoing basis. If some of this sounds completely foreign to you, don't worry. It was to me, too. The most important thing is that it works!

Dr. Torres told me that I might feel sick again after the autologous dendritic cells were received back into my body. My dendritic cells were to be injected subcutaneously, where they would be whisked into my lymphatic system. This was the place they were most likely to come into contact with the cancer cells to which they had been sensitized in the lab.

I was so excited about getting my cells back that I had a hard time settling down and sleeping Wednesday night. "Get into my body!" I almost chanted to myself. I felt like I could sense their excitement about returning to my body/their home, too, as well as my own eager anticipation.

Let me stop at this point and clarify something about not having had a biopsy done. My MD Anderson surgeon had told me she could not conclusively diagnose me with breast cancer unless I had a biopsy. She has reiterated this, months into my healing journey, telling me that she had not yet diagnosed me through biopsy.

Some of you may wonder if I really had breast cancer at all, given that I never have had a biopsy, even to this day.

When the blood that had been drawn to prepare my cancer vaccines was taken to the lab, they performed a cell count of all the various macrophages (lymphocytes, leukocytes, mononuclear cells, monocytes CD14+ or cells which can differentiate into dendritic cells, and CD culture or other leukocytes in other stages of differentiation). They also performed a cell count of the circulating malignant cells. This is not a smoking gun, however, as we all have circulating cancer cells in our bodies at various times. Cancer cells are cells with mutations that keep the cells from experiencing apoptosis (natural programmed cell death). They also begin to multiply extremely rapidly and can invade other body tissues once they form tumors. Only specific mutations allow certain cancer cells to become tumor cells and anchor in an organ or another part of the body, create their own blood flow where they begin to multiply, and create a malignant tumor.

This is where things get interesting. And this is also where medical science is advancing in a very positive way in the cancer-fighting process. Researchers have developed a blood test, referred to as a "liquid biopsy," to diagnose various types of cancers and in order to avoid the risks associated not only with the initial biopsy but also with repeat biopsies. This test is the tDNA/tNOX test. This lab test allows the doctors to know the pathology of the tumor and even the part of the body where the tumor is located with high accuracy. It is extremely helpful to monitor the progress of any malignancy during whatever kind of treatment one would choose to have. It is not yet available to the public but is only being used in studies in the US at the present time; however, even as I write about this, other types of blood biopsy tests are being developed and will be available soon to the public.

There is currently a blood biopsy test used at the Research Genetic Cancer Center (RGCC) in Greece called OncoStat Plus, or the Greek Test. You can ask an integrative medicine or alternative healthcare doctor to order this lab kit and send the frozen plasma to Greece for testing where CTCs and CSCs (cancer stem cells) are isolated, counted, and tested to see what natural substances your particular tumor cells are vulnerable to, as well as which targeted cytotoxic therapies (chemotherapy) might have the strongest impact on them.

In my case, the lab test performed did show definitive evidence of CTCs and billions of "daughter" cells (cancer cells that have not mutated to be able to seed new tumors). The specific cancer cells present in my blood were CD44+ daughter cells, CD44+CD24- daughter cells, and CD44+CD24- circulating tumor cells. The circulating tumor cells are the ones that allowed the breast cancer that had been growing in my breast to metastasize to my lymph node.

So, although I did not have a biopsy performed, the Bi-Rads 5 scores that all my diagnostic imaging had returned were accurate in predicting that the mass and node were highly likely to be malignant. Dr. Kelly's eagle eyes had been correct when he saw this mass and pegged it for breast cancer.

Thursday rolled around, and I was ready. After talking with Dr. Mohammad, researching the topic of intra-tumoral injections on the National Institute of Health website, and checking in with my own intuition, I decided to receive the autologous LAK/NK intra-tumoral injection, so I let them know to "bring it on."

By mid-afternoon, the lab technician delivered my LAK and NK cells. Dr. Torres and the nurse came to my room to connect the lovely bag of bright red, highly oxygenated fluid to my catheter. Before the bag was hooked up to the stand, I asked to hold it for a moment, so I could pray over the life-giving liquid inside. Then I sat back in my recliner and waited to see what would happen as the flow of this precious infusion began.

Within about five minutes, I felt the back of my throat becoming scratchy. It went from scratchy to downright sore in a few more minutes, with my tonsils beginning to swell. Then I felt achy all over, like I was starting to run a fever. We checked, and I did have a low-grade temperature. The immune cells were working! It seemed to me as if they were summoning the rest of the gang to get in there and clean up the damaged cells. I could not have been happier to feel sick.

It only took ten minutes or so for the infusion to be complete. Dr. Torres and the nurse quietly left, and I moved to the bed to sleep. The rest of the day, I stayed quietly in bed, taking it easy and envisioning my hero cells doing what they were there to do. I had prepared a visualization that I focused on during this time.

I was imagining the tumor was a bowl full of birdseed. The immune cells were the birds coming to the bowl to feast on the seeds. If any of the birdseeds fell out of the bowl, other birds would swoop in and gather them from the ground. To help me focus more clearly on this visualization, I thought maybe there would be a YouTube video of birds eating at a bird feeder. I searched and found "Beautiful Birds Singing and Chirping on The Big Red Tea Cup Bird Feeder." I watched it over and over, imagining the cancer cells were the seeds in that big red teacup, and my immune cells were the beautiful little birds feeding from the cup. Having the video to actually watch made my own visualization more focused and even stronger.

By the next morning, the immune response had faded, and I was once again feeling great. I was ready for the amazingly wonderful dendritic cells to "Get into my body!" This was going to be a more intense procedure. Since the injection was going into my upper thigh, I needed to have the area iced down before receiving a shot of lidocaine and then this mighty injection containing my dendritic cells. These dendritic cells are the antigen-producing cells of the immune system. They roam the body like little octopuses, touching with their tentacles all the "not-self" cells and molecules in the body. Depending on what they come in contact with, they use signaling proteins to notify and summon the appropriate immune cells to the site to take care of the intruder. Since these particular cells coming into my body had been sensitized to my specific cancer cells, they would be on the prowl, looking for more of them.

Remember that I called them my pit bull cells? Let the pit bulls loose!

This time the immunologist herself came to administer the vaccine and the intra-tumoral injection. What a process it was to get ready for the injection in my thigh. I was feeling so excited and antsy at the same time. While the immunologist was preparing the injection site with lidocaine, she also prepared the intra-tumoral site. Using topical lidocaine to numb my skin over the tumor, she then did a shallow injection of lidocaine to make the intra-tumoral injection more comfortable.

Yowzer! If that was the more comfortable technique, I would have really hated to have not gotten the lidocaine. Since there was only one nodule of the tumor that was very close to the surface (it actually formed a visible bump under my skin), she injected that nodule on three sides with a bit of the autologous vaccine. I think I was able to relax as much as I did due to my focus on the imagery I had of the cells going straight into the tumor to begin helping the cancer cells transition. I had the sense that the cancer cells were literally stuck in their life cycle. They really needed help to move on, and these LAK and NK cells were on the scene to help out.

Next came the amazing part. As if all of this wasn't amazing enough already, right?

Dr. Torres explained that after the injection to my thigh, I would need to sit still for ten minutes with ice on the injection site, and then I would need to get up and walk briskly for 15 minutes so the cells would be whisked into the lymphatic system. They would migrate throughout the body specifically looking for cancer cells, both daughter cells and circulating tumor cells. After that, I could go back to relaxing, meditating, and visualizing.

Okay, let's do it. I was ready. Before the immunologist filled her syringe with the fluid in the bag, I once again held the bag in my hand, praying over it. I handed the bag back to her, so she could prepare the injection.

Yeeeouch! Oh, my! That was certainly intense. She injected 10 cc of fluid into my thigh. That's a lot! The numbing injection helped immensely, but I was only too happy to sit still for ten minutes and hold the ice bag on my leg. They made sure I was all set, and then left me to my own devices.

After the ten minutes passed, I got up and started to walk briskly in my tiny room. I had not wanted to dress after the intra-tumoral injection since that would have been even more uncomfortable, so I did not feel like I wanted to go walk up and down the hallway in my hospital gown. Not so much. I had a little route around the bed, out to the door, back around the bed, over to the bathroom, into the bathroom, out of the bathroom, and back around the bed. I walked briskly, but it got pretty boring after about two minutes.

I decided to say an affirmation to myself in the bathroom mirror when I went in and out of that tiny room, so the next time I was facing the mirror, I pointed to myself and said, "You are amazing!" Ah, that felt really good. The next time, I said, "You are courageous!" Yes, that was true, and it felt great to hear it out loud. The third time, I said, "You rock my socks!" That felt so good that I just started chanting different affirmations all around the room for the rest of the 15 minutes while pumping my fists in the air to punctuate the positive statements.

The time ended with me on an absolute high emotionally. I was completely ready for healing and completely energized.

When I stopped walking and returned to bed, I realized that my throat was once again becoming a little sore. Not knowing if it was because of the chanting or an immune response, I waited. Yes, starting to feel a little bit achy. Another immune response. Not a very big one, but something was definitely happening.

What a day! I can still feel the energy of that day even now as I write about it. I truly felt like one of Dr. Siegel's extraordinary patients. It was really something else.

Saturday arrived—the going-home day. The first thing I did when I got up was to check the lump to see if there was any difference in how it felt.

Time stood still.

It was actually noticeably smaller.

Noticeably smaller! Already!

The nurse came in after breakfast to remove the IV catheter, and Dr. Torres performed the exam for my release. His eyebrows shot up when he palpated the mass. It was definitely smaller. "You're going to be fine," he said with a big smile.

Before I went downstairs to the car waiting to drive me back into California, the immunologist delivered both a cooler with dry ice containing my frozen autologous dendritic cells and an insulated tote bag with freezer packs and two containers with six vials each of the autologous cytokines. These two packages were more precious than gold to me.

Whew! What a week. And then it was off to Santa Barbara to learn more about why I developed cancer in the first place and how the Issels' protocol would support my continued healing.

AT THE ISSELS
MEDICAL CENTER

Beth

Since this treatment was done with my own cells, and there was no concern about any kind of rejection response, I had the weekend to rest on my own and prepare for my three-week treatment at the Issels Center in Santa Barbara. The apartment I stayed in was overlooking the bay with immediate beach access. It was a beautiful environment in which to focus on healing and to learn a new normal for my life.

The first night at the Issels apartment above the ocean, I was really shocked by the bright yellow light bulbs in the light fixtures and lamps. I made a mental note to pick up some soft white bulbs at the store when I bought my groceries. Later while reading some of the clinic's welcome materials left in the apartment, I learned these yellow light bulbs were strategically placed. Melatonin, a hormone excreted mainly by our pineal glands according to the body's circadian rhythm, can weaken cancer cells. The body's melatonin production is suppressed by using soft white lights with blue light frequency and by watching TV or using the computer right up to the time you go to sleep, again due to the blue light frequency. We don't want to suppress the body's natural melatonin production. I learned that part of my treatment for these three weeks included keeping lights off as it grew dark outside. I came to really enjoy this rhythm, too, and went to bed between 8:30 and 9:00 pm each night. That made it really easy to get up before sunrise so I could watch the sun come up over the mountains ringing the bay and practice my qigong movements. It also gave me the time I wanted to have in order to do my early morning contemplative prayer and meditation.

Qigong Master Chunyi Lin has a guided meditation available on his Spring Forest Qigong website entitled "Cancer Healing Meditation." I downloaded that meditation and started and ended each day with it. In this meditation, Master Lin leads the meditator to an inward focus of healing at the cellular level. I found this guided meditation to be crucial to my ability to stay focused throughout the day and have recommended it to many other newly-diagnosed cancer healers, too. It is available online at www.SpringForestQigong.com.

There is a section in this particular guided meditation where Master Lin says, "You don't need to be afraid of cancer. It is just energy. It is just energy in a form your body doesn't need. You can transform that energy. You are transforming that energy. You are doing it right now." I believe he is right when he says that cancer is just energy. Actually, every cell, every molecule, and every sub-atomic particle in my body is just energy. And the flow of that energy can be directed and transformed by my conscious thoughts.

While in Mexico, I had spent a lot of time journaling, thinking deeply about how my immune system may have become suppressed enough to have allowed not only a malignant tumor but also a metastasis to develop in my body. The hospital had given me a copy of Dr. Josef Issels' (the father of my naturopathic doctor, Dr. Christian Issels) book, *Cancer: A Second Opinion*, to read while I was there. There was so much in that book that spoke to me.

Dr. Josef Issels taught over 50 years ago that the tumor is not where one should focus medical intervention when approaching cancer. It is the entire environment of the body that needs to be addressed. In his view, the tumor is actually a symptom, *not* the summation, of the condition. With the invention of the microscope, which allowed for cellular pathology to be studied, suddenly the shift from the whole system of the person to the pathology of the individual cells happened. Dr. Christian Issels and many other integrative physicians take the systemic approach to healing cancer. I had seen this to be a valid and extremely effective approach during Ivan's prostate-cancer healing process. As his doctors took the systemic approach, the tumor gradually dissipated.

On Monday, my time with Dr. Christian Issels (Dr. Issels) commenced, and he got busy searching for the systemic weaknesses in my body so they could be corrected during my treatment in Santa Barbara to detox and rebuild my health.

I was instructed to head straight to the lab to have more blood drawn before coming to the office for my first day of treatments. The technicians at the lab took 19 vials of my blood! Dr. Issels had ordered all kinds of tests. In order to recommend the right nutritional supplements based on my own body chemistry, he needed a lot of information, and the blood test results were going to give him that.

While I made my way from the lab to the clinic, I was curious about what the office would be like. When I got to the address, the first thing that struck me was how cute the building was. As a matter of fact, all of downtown Santa Barbara with its Mission Revival style of architecture is pretty. And the abundance of flowers sweetly perfumed the air. I felt really happy to be there.

When I first came in, I was given a huge water jug filled with filtered, negatively charged water and told I would need to drink all that water within two days. I started my treatment by meeting Dr. Issels and taking a seat across from his desk in his private office. He used two biofeedback scans to gather more information about my body chemistry and areas of stress. He asked me a lot of questions, which I answered willingly, even adding details he had not asked for.

Then he stopped.

"Have you always been an over achiever?" he asked.

"Why, yes, I believe I have been," was my quick response.

I'll get back to that exchange between us in a bit because it's an important piece of the treatment process.

After my thorough intake appointment with Dr. Issels, I went on to meet with Dr. Walter Kim, who is a nuclear radiologist and has been working with Dr. Issels for the past nine years. He reviewed my previous diagnostic scans and the lab reports from the Issels ImmunoOncology Hospital, and he told me what he was looking for with the labs I had just had my blood drawn for. He shared with me that all the immune therapies I would be doing at the Issels Clinic were geared to optimize my immune system and weaken the cancerous tumor cells in my body. He told me that they did expect the tumor to continue to shrink and the lymph node to normalize. He was glad to hear that I had already made an appointment with Dr. Kelly to be re-scanned with ultrasound immediately following my three weeks with them.

Next, I was introduced to the nurses in the IV lounge and told to choose a comfortable recliner and get ready to have a new catheter inserted. I would have this catheter in for the next three days to make it easier on my system to receive the multiple IV infusions I would be having each day.

Each day was slightly different, but a definite pattern emerged. I would arrive at the center in the morning, either go into the IV lounge for my infusions or have one of the other natural treatments first. Several times per week, I had acupuncture, oxygen therapy, infrared sauna therapy, two kinds of cellular stimulation done with energetic electrical frequencies, colon hydrotherapy, psychotherapy, and massage. I was not able to lie in the hyperbaric chamber to receive hyperbaric therapy due to the fact that I could not equalize my ears in the prone position. I needed to sit up, but the inflatable pods would not allow for that, so the oxygen therapy I got while at the center was not done under pressure.

Every day we received a salad and soup for lunch, liquid minerals, and a small cup of vitamins. Dr. Issels prescribed other supplements for me that I took back to the apartment. We also had guest speakers who would come in during the lunch hour to address topics like eating and nutrition, hydrating properly, and guided meditation.

The Issels protocol includes following a ketogenic diet. A ketogenic diet causes the body to burn ketones for energy, instead of glucose. Since cancer prefers sugar as an energy source, restricting sugar is thought to weaken cancer cells. Mutated cells do not have the ability to burn ketones while our normal cells do. While the Misner Plan leans one toward ketosis, it is not primarily a ketogenic diet. Getting the body into ketosis requires that you severely restrict your carbohydrate calories. Dr. Issels' recommendation is no more than 50 net carb grams per day while healing cancer. That means if something contains 15 grams of carbs per serving, but it also has four grams of fiber, you get to deduct the fiber grams from the carb grams to arrive at the net carb intake for that food serving.

There are many good reasons for putting the body into ketosis while healing cancer, not the least of which is restricting the fuel that cancer cells require for their survival: sugars. So I began to follow a ketogenic version of the Misner Plan: 80% of my daily caloric intake came from healthy fats. I restricted my intake of simple carbohydrates, ate only organically grown fruits and vegetables, and ate no dairy products, other than a very small amount of goat cheese and yogurt. I counted net carb grams, keeping them fewer than 50 grams per day, and I ate only eggs and small fish (sardines, mackerel, and anchovies) as my animal protein sources, and then only rarely did I have animal protein.

The most enjoyable of all the treatments for me were the sessions with Dr. Revel Miller, the psychotherapist. I told him the first time I met him that he would be the centerpiece for my treatment, and I meant that. I asked to add extra sessions with him to my treatment package because I knew that I needed his particular expertise to be sure I did not go home and repeat the destructive pattern of taking on so much that I ended up suppressing my immune system again from stress. His mantra to me, over the three weeks and upon my release, was: "Beth, no stress—*none*—for six months during your treatment."

It was through my work with him that I began to view the tumor as a tiny messenger arriving with a very important message for me to which I must pay heed. I did not want to feel like this tiny messenger was an enemy. This tissue was, after all, my tissue, my cells, just damaged and needing help to transition and move on. Even though I am a martial artist, and it would have been easy to go to war, I did not want to use a warfare motif: fighting cancer, being strong in the battle, gaining the upper hand—no, none of that. I chose phrases that are gentle and positive: healing cancer, helping these cells transform, listening to the tiny messenger, loving my cells, and helping them become unstuck.

Later, I will go more into the work Dr. Miller and I did together, as well as counseling I would receive later at home, but I'll just say here that I was correct about his part of the process being the center of my healing work at the Issels Clinic. I really enjoyed the new rhythm of my gentle treatment and leaned into my time there to easily heal, rest, recalibrate, and center deeply inward.

As my treatment time passed, I began to make friends with some of the other patients, and I'm in touch with them still today. I came to have favorites among the nurses and even wrote a poem for one of them. I remembered while having my treatments that I used to write poetry and songs. I've even had two poems published in two different anthologies of poetry. Writing poems is one of my favorite things to do. It is relaxing and gives me an outlet for expressing my emotions. Through this process, I rediscovered this interest. I enjoyed writing poems about the smallest things, and I'm putting them in a book to be released later on.

Each day at Issels, I received three different types of infusions. Most of the infusions were targeted to detox and rebuild my immune system. Some of the infusions were specifically targeted to weaken any cells with DNA mutations that might be in my body. I also received auto-hemotherapy, an injection of my own blood cells into the muscle tissue. This allows the lymphatic system to get immediate, current information about what proteins are being released into my blood stream from pathogens, including cancer cells, so they may summon the appropriate immune cells to correct any problems. It is a real-time vaccine for any pathogens present. Simple and brilliant!

Another infusion I should have received would have been curcumin, the chemical component in turmeric, which is renowned for its anti-inflammatory properties. The skin test done the day before I was to receive the curcumin infusion revealed that I am actually allergic to it. This was very interesting to learn, as I had been consuming turmeric regularly in my diet. Upon learning this, I cut it out, and then I noticed not long afterwards that the severe pain in my left foot which I'd had for a couple of years faded and disappeared completely. A couple of months later, I began to have "Golden Milk," an Ayurvedic drink rich in turmeric, which gives it a bright gold color. Within three days, the intense pain in that foot returned, only to disappear for good when I stopped having that drink.

So, even though turmeric is a potent anti-oxidant with powerful anti-inflammatory properties, it has not been part of my immune therapy. When healing from something as serious as cancer, it is important to avoid any and all allergens, so being tested for food allergies is really critical. If a curcumin allergy is not a concern, it can be a valuable inclusion in a treatment protocol. It is a common enough allergen, though, that the Issels Center tests every patient before administering any curcumin infusions.

Another aspect of the Issels' immune therapy included colon hydrotherapy, about which I knew very little at the time. My experiences with the colon hydrotherapist, who was located a couple of blocks away, were very positive, and I have continued with the practice beyond my time in Santa Barbara. Since my treatment package included a minimal number of treatments, I requested to add the optimal number of treatments and went more frequently. The colon hydrotherapist also did coffee enemas during the colonics treatment, which is thought to stimulate glutathione production in the liver. Glutathione is a peptide that helps our bodies fight cancer by supporting the detox pathway responsible for reducing carcinogens and their negative impact.

Having been a chiropractic patient since I was ten years old, I found a really wonderful chiropractor next door to the clinic, and I did weekly spinal adjustments with him to support the immune therapy I was receiving. Although not a part of the Issels' protocol, I wanted to be sure this healing modality was part of my healing path.

Ivan and I have several good friends who live in the Santa Barbara area, and one of them in particular, Dawa Tarchin Phillips, made a point to stay in close contact with me. Among other things, Dawa leads a local Buddhist sangha and is a classically trained Tibetan monk. He also speaks some of the same languages I do: English, French, and German. We met for regular conversations about my spiritual life, and he gave me some thought-provoking spiritual exercises to do, as well as certain inquiries to hold space for as I did my contemplative work. These conversations were deeply meaningful to me and brought me closer to God as I experienced a more profound, divine connection with the Creator.

During my sessions with Dawa, I realized that I wanted to lean more fully into the meaning of my given name: Elisabeth. Elisabeth means "house of God" in Hebrew. I shortened my name after college to Beth as a way to more easily answer the phone for the chiropractic office where I worked. Try saying, "Good morning. Dr. Dorothy's office. This is Elisabeth," a hundred times per day. It's not easy. Shortening Elisabeth to Beth made that much simpler. What came to my mind during my healing time was that Elisabeth has a very deep meaning. While Beth can be just any old house, Elisabeth is God's house, and that is who I am.

Another aspect of my healing process included alpaca therapy. Yes, you read that correctly. I have a dear friend who lives on an alpaca ranch outside of Ventura, California. It was a short 35-minute drive south from where I was staying, so I made plans for the second weekend of my Santa Barbara visit to drive out to meet the herd. Many clinical studies have shown that having pets or being around animals can raise our immune function. I don't currently have any pets due to the amount of travel Ivan and I do with our company, BNI. And I have wanted to meet the alpacas ever since Tracy started raising them. They hold a certain fascination for me.

I was not disappointed when I spent time with the herd. We went into one of the pens with the females and put down yoga mats. Slowly, the more curious girls made their way over to investigate whether or not we had treats for them. Once they became comfortable with our presence, a couple of them actually rested beside our mats under the big shade tree we were under. It was wonderful! I know for sure my brain released a lot of neurotransmitters that told my body, "All is well. Keep all systems running right now. There are no threats to your existence."

The third weekend I was there, I felt ready for some social time, so I accepted an invitation from two of my girlfriends who live in Santa Barbara, Aranza and Inga, to meet at the farmer's market and then go to brunch. I enjoyed being with my friends very much—it filled my heart! But the noise at the market and again at the restaurant were overwhelming to me. I had been isolated more or less for about three weeks by this point (one week in the hospital and two weeks at the clinic), and I was not used to being in crowds. I found it difficult to keep my calm center with all the hubbub around me. That made me wonder what my experience would be like coming out of my Healing Bubble and re-engaging with my and Ivan's normal travel schedule and public appearances, where we would be in the midst of anywhere between 200 and 2000 people at a time.

For the last week of the Issels' detox and rebuild program, I moved to a small house located a few blocks from the clinic so I could walk back and forth for my daily treatments. I wanted to leave my rental car parked and simplify my days. The little house I rented had two apartments, and I took the apartment in the back with a large deck that opened onto a Zen garden with edible plants I could harvest and prepare with my meals. It was lovely.

It was during my last week of treatment that I did the genomic test to evaluate the genes regulating my body's detoxification processes. Dr. Issels has learned (as did his father before him) that most cancer patients have some genetic mutations involving the body's two detox pathways. I received the results of this testing after I had returned home, and I learned that I have seven mutations in these pathways, as well as one gene missing completely. The missing gene is one of the three genes that regulate the body's glutathione production, and one of the other two genes in this group is mutated. I only have one gene that is giving my body the proper blueprint for glutathione production. Since glutathione is a powerful substance, critical to detoxification, normal carcinogens are doubly carcinogenic to me. Things like pesticides, smog, cigarette smoke, and the like, are twice as toxic in my body as they are in a person with all three of their genes intact.

So having this test performed was a very important element to my subsequent healing process, as well as knowing what preventative measures I need to take to support my specific body with its mutations. I now know that I need to supplement with glutathione for the rest of my life. In the meantime, I continued to receive glutathione infusions at the Issels clinic. It also means that coffee enemas are very important for my continued health. I will explain more about this a little bit later in my story.

Finally, it was time to pick Ivan up from the airport. He flew in to Santa Barbara to be with me for the last couple of days of my treatment and to drive me to Pasadena for my follow-up ultrasound scan. It was so wonderful to be back together with him. I had done a lot of introspection and enjoyed having time to reconnect with myself, but then it was time to re-enter the space being a couple takes up in life, and I cannot tell you how utterly delicious it was to have him close.

On my last day at the Issels Clinic, Ivan went with me to sit down with Dr. Kim to get my going-home orders and learn what my home therapy was going to look like as I continued the Issels immune therapy in Austin. I brought with me a small list of questions. Dr. Kim had been so patient with me all along with the myriad of questions I brought into his office every few days, but I'm sure the short list was appreciated by him.

He recommended that I take two prescriptions away with me: one for low-dose Naltrexone (LDN) and one for Metformin to keep my blood sugar low (remember, cancer prefers sugar). I accepted the LDN prescription, but I knew that I was able to keep my own blood sugar low by remaining in ketosis, so I declined the Metformin. The side effects that come along with this medication were not desirable, and I knew I had the discipline to eat in a way that would not give cancer cells their preferred energy source.

Just before checking out, the nurse prepared my final injection: the precious bag of dendritic cells that had traveled with me from Mexico. Once again, I was eager for them to "Get in my body!"

The front desk staff put together my package of recommended supplements, and I returned my drinking water jug. My time at the clinic had come to an end. I was ready to get home in order to anchor my gentle healing process and to create the Healing Bubble in Austin I needed to maintain during my time of home therapy.

MEASURABLE RESULTS

Ivan

Taking Elisabeth to Pasadena for the ultrasound scan in order to see whether the immune therapies were having the desired impact was both exciting and tense. I felt very supportive of her choice of treatment, but there was an element of suspense for me. Even though I had been through the natural healing process twice before, I am a guy that likes data, graphs, and charts to verify that a treatment process is working. This scan would be the beginnings of a graph on which we could plot the changes to the size of the tumor.

We spent Sunday night at a hotel just a block from Dr. Kelly's office. After a nervous breakfast, we walked together, hand in hand, to the office. Elisabeth was so certain the scan would show an improvement that when she saw Dr. Kelly, she pumped both her fists in the air like she had just won the prize fight.

"Let's see what I did!" she exulted to the doctor.

I like to be a little bit more guarded and quietly anticipate good news. Not Elisabeth. She calls it in!

Literally, sometimes.

As Elisabeth prepared for the scan, I tried to encourage her to stay positive even if the scan was not as good as she was hoping for it to be, just in case things had not gone in the direction she was anticipating. I reminded her that it had taken several months for my scans to begin showing improvement. I really did not want her to be disappointed if her healing was going more slowly than she wanted. She just smiled wanly at me and called out to the nurse that she was ready for Dr. Kelly to start the scan.

Dr. Kelly and his technician entered the room and dimmed the lights, so we could all see the monitor clearly. Dr. Kelly's technician started the scan with Dr. Kelly instructing her where to place the transducer. The mass swam into view. I could tell by the quick, quiet intake of Elisabeth's breath that she was disappointed to see it was still there. I squeezed her hand in reassurance.

"Hmmm," Dr. Kelly said. "Move down a little," he said to the tech.

After viewing the tumor from many angles and having the tech take measurements, he asked her to move over to the lymph node.

"Look at this," he said to us, pointing to the monitor. There was a faint, hazy white halo in the middle of the node. "This is where the hilum is starting to be visible again."

"That's good, right?" Elisabeth eagerly asked.

"Oh yes, very good. It is showing signs of recovering." Dr. Kelly replied with a smile.

Elisabeth beamed. She shot me a glance that said, "You see?" I could not help but smile because of her indomitable spirit.

When Dr. Kelly was done with the exam and had captured all the images he wanted to, he turned to us and said, "Well, the tumor is smaller and there is less cancer. The lymph node is looking better, too. You are on the right track. Keep talking to your cells."

This time, Elisabeth looked at me with a funny expression that held both relief and excitement at the same time. Then she shouted, and we high-fived each other. Dr. Kelly was all smiles and invited us to join him in his office to take a closer look at the images.

After Elisabeth dressed, we met Dr. Kelly in his office. She hugged him right away. Then we sat down so he could explain what we had seen. He compared the images from a month prior with the images from this appointment. It was clear that the mass was both more lightly colored on the scan and a bit smaller. When he showed us the images from the color Doppler imaging, he pointed out that there was still a certain amount of blood flow to the mass, indicating that the tumor was still angiogenic.

Even that could not deflate Elisabeth.

Elisabeth then asked Dr. Kelly what he would have expected to see on the scan if a patient had not done chemotherapy for a month. She wanted to know if it could have been expected that a tumor and lymph node might have been able to show this kind of improvement without the standard of care: chemotherapy. He told her that he would fully expect the mass to be larger, darker, and that there would be more metastatic lymph nodes if the patient had done no chemotherapy in the month between scans.

She was so happy and so excited that there was measurable improvement that she just about floated back to the hotel to pack up and return to the airport. Every half hour or so, she would grab my shirtsleeve and gently pull on it and smile up at me with excitement. I shared in her excitement, although probably more guardedly. She still had quite a ways to go in order to have a clean bill of health.

But the healing was obviously and irrefutably underway.

CLEARING OUT THE OLD

Beth

Many natural healthcare practitioners find that healing starts in the gut where a large part of our digestive process and immune function takes place. Any compromise in this area can lead to malnourishment and compromised immune function, neither of which lead one to health. Although I (Beth) did not understand at the time why the Issels protocol included colon hydrotherapy or colonics, which can be connected to improved gut health, I had made an appointment with the wonderful colon hydrotherapist referred by the Issels clinic. Her office was only a few blocks away, so I walked myself straight over there on my second day of treatment.

I entered her suite with a little trepidation and a lot of curiosity. I had taken two colonics treatments in the past. To be honest, I was not a big fan. Both of the sessions I had done previously were done by a colon hydrotherapy machine, which means that the water used to hydrate my colon was delivered under pressure. When I felt the need to eliminate, the therapist turned off the fill and allowed nature to take its course. The therapist recommended by the Issels Clinic allows the fills to be done by gravity. The tank was mounted about two feet above the treatment table on the wall. This allowed for a much gentler treatment.

She started my first treatment by giving me a few gentle fills to evacuate the sigmoid colon of the hard, solid, dehydrated stool that would have made my first coffee enema difficult. After that, she did a fill with about 2 cups of a special type of coffee designed specifically for this purpose. She set a timer for 15 minutes and asked me to hold the coffee, if I could. There were a couple of moments during the 15 minutes that I took some long, deep breaths in order to hold the coffee, although I still did not understand why a coffee fill was important for healing my body.

After the coffee enema, she spent the next 30 minutes flushing out my colon. A couple of times she did a small fill with chlorophyll. When I asked her why she used chlorophyll, she let me know that it helps to reduce any gas trapped in my gut. During colon hydrotherapy, reducing discomfort caused by gas is a very good thing.

I could not believe the amount of waste my body was releasing. As the release continued, she was watching the evacuation tube and told me that a lot of hard, dark, old crud was leaving my system. When I asked her how often I should do this treatment, she suggested five sessions in a row, followed by three times a week for the rest of the time I was in Santa Barbara. I happily booked sessions with her for Wednesday through Saturday.

For the rest of the week, my body continued to release a shocking amount of old, putrid waste each time I had a session. It was not until Saturday that it felt like my system was finally where it should be, and I began to feel lighter and clearer. I also began to research and study the health benefits of both colon hydrotherapy and coffee enemas.

I learned that when solid waste is held longer than it should be in the large intestine due to weak colon muscles or constipation induced by eating the wrong kinds of foods or by being dehydrated, some of the toxins (such as heavy metals, dangerous hormones, and chemicals) that are meant to be released through the stool are actually reabsorbed into the body through the rectal veins, from which they pass back through the liver. Recycling these toxins can actually overload the liver, which is usually very busy purifying the blood from even more of these toxins. In the case of someone who wants to support the immune system (like me, during my quest to reverse cancer naturally), this is critical. It is so vital to health that I have continued with colon hydrotherapy and coffee enemas while back home in Texas. I'll say more about that in a bit.

So, why specifically are coffee enemas so important? What I learned is that coffee, especially the type of coffee produced for coffee enemas, such as S. A. Wilson's Gold, powerfully supports the liver's detoxification process. Coffee contains palmitic acid (highest in green coffee beans), which was linked to higher immune function in a 1982 *in vivo* study at the University of Southern Florida and University of Boston on the ability of green coffee beans to effect a substantial increase in glutathione production. Glutathione is a peptide so critical to health relating to cancer that it is often administered intravenously prior to chemotherapy treatments in traditional cancer care. Most alternative care cancer centers use IV glutathione as a course of therapy to support the detoxification process in order to reduce the negative impact of carcinogenic substances in the body.

A reduced level of this critical peptide, in conjunction with my suppressed immune function, is one of the main factors I believe led to my development of a malignant tumor. Remember that after having a genetic test done to check for genetic mutations in my detox pathways, I learned that of the three genes that regulate the body's production of this critical enzyme, one is intact, one is mutated, and one is missing completely. Now that I know this, I believe it is even more critical to my continued health that I make coffee enemas and colon hydrotherapy a lifelong part of my healthy practices.

Before I returned home to Texas, I found a colon hydrotherapist in my hometown who also does gravity colonics, and I made an appointment with her for my first week back from California. When I showed up at her clinic for my first appointment, she surprised me by asking if I had brought my colon-hydrotherapy prescription with me.

"My prescription?" I asked incredulously. Wait, isn't this Texas, the land of the *free*? Nope, not when it comes to the dastardly colon hydrotherapy. One must indeed have a prescription from a medical practitioner in order to receive colon hydrotherapy in our state. You can open-carry a gun without a license, but you cannot book colonics treatment without a doctor's approval and prescription.

Then I got my second surprise during the treatment when I asked her if she could do a coffee enema during my session. "I cannot insert anything other than pure water into your colon," she replied.

"No chlorophyll?" I asked.

"Nope," she replied. "No chlorophyll. No coffee. Just pure water."

Wow.

After that session, I learned more about how to perform colon hydrotherapy for myself at home—on YouTube. It is not rocket science, folks. I began to do regular enemas, working my way up to filling with three to four cups of filtered water, chlorophyll as needed (powdered Sun Chlorella mixed with six ounces of filtered water), holding that for up to ten minutes, then releasing. I also worked my way up to two rounds of holding two cups of S. A. Wilsons' coffee at a time for 15 minutes in succession. I did coffee enemas three times per week during my healing phase.

In order to truly do colon hydrotherapy, I purchased an enema bucket that holds 2½ quarts of filtered water so I can fill my colon with five quarts of warm water during the course of my own treatment. I fill my colon until I feel a strong need to eliminate. I release and then fill again. I continue do colon hydrotherapy once a week, and I include two coffee fills to boost immune function.

Here are a couple of links to get more information about coffee enemas and their health benefits:

http://sawilsons.com/library/basic-coffee-enema-procedure-and-recipe/

https://draxe.com/coffee-enema/

Here are the main take-aways about this subject:

- Colon hydrotherapy can be an important part of the body's detoxification process and when done regularly, may help us stay healthier.

- Colonic treatments may help us avoid recycling toxins into the liver from stagnant or impacted fecal matter that is meant for faster evacuation than is normally happening for most of us.

- When we do coffee enemas, the palmitic acid in coffee may help us produce more glutathione, an enzyme that is critical to our detoxification process.

- The caffeine in special green coffee produced for coffee enemas, like S. A. Wilson's Gold, may help the liver's detoxification processes.

- Check your state's laws concerning colon hydrotherapy. You may be required to have a prescription from an MD, DO, or ND in order to book a colonics treatment from a colon hydrotherapist.

HEALING THE BODYMIND

Ivan and Beth

When Elisabeth found out that psychotherapy was part of the Issels protocol for healing, she was relieved because she realized that the many of the things that had contributed to her immune system becoming suppressed were psychological in nature. She has always been a very driven person, prone to repeating an intensely busy cycle, punctuated by dips or crashes. I (Ivan) have watched her caught in this repetitive flow for nearly 30 years now. Even she could see that she had let this cycle repeat itself with a vengeance prior to discovering the lump in her breast. Truth be told, any cancer clinic that purports to help patients heal needs to address the psychological component, since so much of what causes the body's immune system to be suppressed can be somatic and traced back to emotional/psychological roots.

Dr. Revel Miller worked with Elisabeth during her time at the Issels Medical Center in Santa Barbara, California, to help her identify where her life had once again gotten overly full. It was mostly relating to her non-profit work. Shortly before moving to Austin, Elisabeth and I had started a new movement within our non-profit, the BNI Foundation, called Business Voices. This movement has been changing the trajectory of the lives of children all over the world as other business owners have become aware of the challenges faced by today's youth and have been investing their time, talent, and treasure in their own communities.

As with starting anything new, it has taken a lot of time and energy on

Elisabeth's part to create the momentum needed to see this concept take hold, not only in our company, BNI, but also in the business world in general. Business Voices was growing, and staffing changes within the foundation made it necessary for Beth to begin running the non-profit for a time, while also serving as Secretary of the Board of Directors for the BNI Foundation and simultaneously conducting the executive search for a new foundation director. Not being a person who goes into anything half-heartedly, as you have already learned about her, Elisabeth really gave up her own personal life to invest in the success of the foundation and to be sure to bring in a foundation director who would be the right person to take things to the next level.

Elisabeth also had a hard time creating harmony over the four or five years preceding her diagnosis. We had just moved from California (where we had lived for decades) to Texas, closed on two homes, moved one of our children with us to Texas and then on to Rhode Island. We lost both of my parents, to whom she was very close, and she nearly lost her father to a surgical accident which is why we relocated to Texas where her parents reside. We moved one more time in Austin from a downtown condo to a home outside of town and set up a part-time vacation condo on the coast of Texas that we also planned to rent out to others. That was a lot of intensive change happening over a short period of time. She literally moved, arranged for packing and transport of the contents of the homes, oversaw offloading and delivery of the contents in several other homes, including a storage facility, unpacked and set up the furniture and belongings of six houses in the space of about two years.

Dr. Miller helped Beth create the right perspective regarding her personal space, boundaries, and self-care. He helped her identify the things she could delegate to others, and then identify who those others were so that she left the Issels Center with a solid game plan. He also emphasized over and over that she could not allow any stress to invade her days for the following six months. He talked about her care-taking mode directed towards me during my prostate-healing process—she now needed to apply that to herself.

There are many people who write and lecture about the variety of emotional causes for immune system suppression. This entire field is quite fascinating and has a very fancy name: psychoneuroimmunology. We like using the simple term BodyMind. There is current, solid research that links emotional states, prolonged stress, and certain traumatic experiences to a negative change in one's immune functions. Dawson Church writes extensively about these connections in his wonderful book about epigenetics, *The Genie in Your Genes*, illustrating and explaining how our emotional states of mind can stimulate the neuropeptides that send the signals to our cells, switching on and off the tumor suppressor genes and oncogenes, even shutting down the entire immune system. Dr. Bernie Siegel also writes about this dynamic in *Love, Medicine, and Miracles*, saying that he often looks backward as many as seven years into his cancer patients' lives to identify a moment of deep grief or loss in order to find the trigger for immune function suppression.

I (Beth) had such a moment of deep grief in 2012, five years before finding this breast tumor. Sometimes we are lucky enough to have that "heart pet" that just finds its way deep, deep within our hearts. I had this in my sweet Coton de Tulear, Coco Belle. I really grieved the loss of this dog and was not able to be in public without sunglasses due to the constant crying I experienced in the weeks after my dog crossed over the "rainbow bridge." Even remembering this loss brings fresh tears and an ache into my heart. I loved her so much, and she adored me back.

Less than a year after Coco Belle's sad death, Ivan's mother died three days before he was diagnosed with cancer (my other Coton de Tulear died the same weekend), and all the other things Ivan mentioned above started to happen, cascading into my life one after the other. It was just too much stress, and I did not have tools to handle it without my immune system becoming suppressed. It's quite possible that the unmanaged stress sent the critical signals to my body to switch off the tumor suppressor genes and switch on the oncogenes, not something I could afford to have happen given my genetic mutations in the detox pathways.

Some people are slow learners. I must be one of them. My friend Cherie says that there are no slow learners—just thorough ones. That's me: a thorough learner! Especially when it comes to avoiding the Overload Syndrome (OS).

My first experience with OS was way, way, way back in my 20s. I was working with a psychotherapist at that time to get help for clinical depression and a lot of anxiety. He gave me an assignment at the beginning of our work together. The assignment was to write down everything I had to do for three days in the order I did them. If I multi-tasked, he wanted me to write each thing beside the other(s) in the same time slot.

When I came back the next week to review my assignment with him, he nearly fell off his chair. "You need about nine people's days to tackle what you are trying to tackle in just one day of the one life you have been given," he admonished me.

He helped me to untangle my to-do list and make only the commitments that I could keep at that point in my life, while still leaving room for things I did simply because I enjoyed them. I came to see that my depression and anxiety were self-inflicted.

But I did not learn my lesson yet.

I repeated the same scenario in my third decade, in my fourth decade, and now, in the opening years of my fifth decade. Except now, the end result of this propensity wasn't depression or anxiety (although they were along for the ride, too). No, the end result has been cancer.

There is a direct link between a lack of self-care and the development of the most serious conditions that arise as a result of a suppressed immune system, and this is why I am writing about this now. Doctors and research studies around the world all agree: stress kills.

I think our digital age makes it even harder to stay in touch with the things our physical bodies need from us. We have become Big Brains, connected to the world online like never before, completely networked into this worldwide, digital brain. And it isn't happening only at work anymore. It's from the moment our eyes fly open to the second they shut tight at the end of the day, even as we are still reading our posts, Pinterest, Instagram, BBC, or whatever it is you read. We are sitting (sometimes even lying) in front of large and small screens for hours, with nothing moving except our eyes and maybe our fingertips—for hours and cumulative days, weeks, months, and years. Some of us (I'll even admit to this) take a mobile device into the bathroom in the middle of the night to see what we may be missing while we take that biological break that woke us up in the first place!

Except that we are not Big Brains, and we certainly are not digital entities, even though we may act like we have lost sight of that version of reality. We are conscious, sentient beings with a physical body that has a direct interface with our minds. And if our physical bodies are not taken care of the way they need to be in order to continue functioning well, life will not turn out for us the way we envision.

I certainly never envisioned I would ever be dealing with the "C" word. I can look back now and see the arrogance of that position. The short list below outlines the most critical ways our body-machines need us to care for them to keep us in the flow of health. This list comes from a lived experience that I hope and pray you never have to go through:

- Move.
- Breathe.
- Hydrate.
- Sleep.

This list is short, but take an honest, hard look at these four things. Are you doing them well? Most of us, myself included before this tiny messenger brought them more to my awareness, are not doing even one of these things well, never mind hitting all of them to the best of our abilities. And yet our health, our bodies, and our very lives depend on them as a group.

Now, it's not reasonable to expect that life will be stress free, because stress is a normal reaction to change, and change is always happening in our lives. But I believe it is possible to reassure the body that the stress we are under is not life-threatening.

Until we adopt specific practices that switch the immune function fully back on, our bodies will not know the difference between the stress of losing a pet and the stress of seeing a truck heading straight for us in a head-on collision. In both cases, our emotions telegraph the body that our existence is in danger, and our bodies shut down all non-essential activities in order to prepare for the life-saving fight or flight.

The immune system is one of those systems that pauses during the fight or flight response, and the shutdown is cued by shallow breathing, tightened muscles pulling your shoulders up to your ears, and a racing heartbeat. Another system that stops during fight or flight is digestion. I believe this is why I could develop cancer even though I was fairly strict with my diet, following our Misner Plan closely.

When Dr. Bill Kellas of the Center for Advanced Medicine was working with me in 2013 to identify why my high C-reactive protein level was so high, my pancreas had also shut down, and lab tests showed that I was not digesting macronutrients—the elements in foods that keep us healthy: fats, proteins, and carbohydrates. I had apparently picked up a virus during one of our international travels that attacked my pancreas. Why? Most likely because my immune system had already dropped its guard and allowed the virus to get established.

So, I needed to learn how to cue my body that all was well—let all these vital systems once again work at full capacity. There was no lion in the shrubs beside me! One of the quickest ways to reset the body's physical response to stress is to breathe deeply. In the words of WildFit founder, Eric Edmeades, breathing deeply simply causes the body to say, "Well, she's breathing calmly, so everything has to be okay."

Check your breathing right now as you read this book. Is there room to deepen the inhale? Can you exhale more completely? What about during the day when you are at work, checking email, in an online meeting, or with a client? If you notice closely, you may find that you are breathing shallowly or even, as I noticed I did frequently, holding your breath. It took me over six months to stop exhaling and then pausing—for a *long* time—before inhaling again.

Imagine a rabbit hiding under a rock, waiting for a coyote to lose interest in the chase. That bunny is breathing very shallowly, or perhaps even holding its breath. You may find yourself falling into that breathing pattern, but your life is not in danger!

So, the easiest way to give your body the "all clear" message is to stop many times in your day to take deep, intentional breaths. Breathing all the way in, filling all the lobes of your lungs (you actually have three lobes in the right lung and two lobes in the left lung), then exhaling completely, creating a full exchange of air in and out of all five of your lung lobes, is one of the best ways to be sure your immune function stays high throughout times of stress. You may also relax your shoulders and gaze calmly out across the horizon. This tells your body that there are no threats. A creature that is relaxed and has the leisure to stand and gaze far out into the distance is not a creature under attack. It sends a powerful signal to the body that all is well.

Another simple technique is the Emotional Freedom Technique (EFT), sometimes called Tapping. Tapping uses ancient, traditional Chinese medicine (TCM) acupuncture points to reset the energy channels of the body that regulate our stress response. Tapping also stimulates the relaxation response. Any time the relaxation response is triggered, our body brings all of the functions back online that it suppresses during times of extended stress. Nick Ortner has a great, four-minute video on YouTube called "How to Tap" with instructions on how to perform EFT.

The Issels protocol in Santa Barbara, California, included sessions with another type of counselor, a hypnotherapist. She worked with the patients using guided meditation to trigger our relaxation responses. She also offered to work individually with the patients being treated to create an audio recording that would support our conscious goals by retraining the subconscious mind once we returned home. So much of our behavior is controlled by the subconscious mind—it is responsible for over 80% of our brain function! And we do not have conscious control of what our subconscious mind is programming our brains to do and think. It became clearer to me that my subconscious had another agenda for me, and I had not been able to end the cycle of creating the overload that was compromising my health and my life. I had already begun to do a lot of amazing work with our good friend Shelly Lefkoe, who uses the Lefkoe Method to help us get to the core of limiting beliefs, and now I was getting the chance to intentionally reprogram my subconscious mind, the part of my brain that was creating behaviors based on beliefs set decades ago that I had not been able to access before this.

Far from using hypnotherapy to do fun parlor tricks and embarrass friends at a dinner party, a great hypnotherapist can help us re-teach our subconscious minds to support our goals, whether they are healing goals, educational goals, or relationship goals.

As the Issels Center brought this information into Elisabeth's awareness, Dr. Miller suggested that I (Ivan) join the two of them for her last counseling session. In this final session, we came up with a metaphor for Beth to use to express when the majority of her day has been focused on the things that nourish her soul, rather than things that drain her. She agreed that a day spent nourishing her spirit would be a day when she was "singing." Once we returned home, it became easy for me to ask her, "Were you singing today?" And it was easy for her to say, "I had a day filled with singing." She also gave me permission to ask her, if I saw her over-engaged in business endeavors in a way that eroded her time for self-care, "Are you singing right now?" We have found in our 29 years of married life together that metaphors like this really work for us, so it was great to have this tactic.

Dr. Miller also encouraged her to continue working with a psychotherapist when she returned home to Austin. Always curious about new and unique things, Elisabeth investigated equine therapy, counseling done in a horse arena with a psychotherapist, a horse, and a horse trainer to interpret the horse's communication via its behaviors. Since horses have always been a part of her "singing," she looked for a therapist at home who specialized in equine therapy.

Finding RED Arena and counselor Lindsey and horse trainer Elisa was simply wonderful. The first session in the pasture, I (Beth) walked around with the ladies and simply observed the herd. I would have the chance to meet the herd up close and choose my equine partner. The first horse I noticed was a gelding who was very alert, moving around the pasture with purpose and energy.

"That's the herd boss," Elisa shared. "A few of the mares are out of the pasture today, getting ready for an event at another barn. He is very aware that the entire herd is not here, and he's watching for them to return."

Herd boss, huh? I was married to a herd boss. My husband manages a herd of 250,000 BNI members as the founder and Chief Visionary Officer (CVO) of our company. It's just the way it is. I decided I wanted to work with a horse that would be less distracted by needing to manage the herd.

I've been around horses nearly all my life, and I love them. They are such emotional and regal creatures, and I know they can also be high-strung and flighty. I have permanent dents in my body to prove that. Two things I had to do to engage with the horses in the herd were very different for me than the way I previously had worked with horses.

Elisa and Lindsey taught me the "red light, green light" game with the herd. If one of the horses continued grazing, or stood still, looking away from me, I was free to continue approaching that horse. The moment that horse lifted its head or turned and looked directly at me, I was to stop. As prey animals, they will always see humans as the predator. When the horse felt comfortable that I was not a threat, and it dropped its head and continued to graze or just looked away, I was okay to move closer. Now, this was uncomfortable for me. I was used to "being the boss" with the horse. I was taught to move boldly, take command—literally to be the boss. I was about to learn a whole new way to interact with my friends, the horses.

As I made this observation aloud to Lindsey, she asked me if it had become my habit to take command of the room when I come into it. I had to admit that it had. She asked me if that caused me to feel any pressure. Again, I had to say yes. Here was an area of life that was causing tension for me that I did not even realize.

Additionally, I had to get a "horse handshake" before I could touch the horse I was approaching. What? A horse handshake? Yes, you read that right. The horse needed to reach its nose to my outstretched hand and give it a sniff. That is the horse handshake. Well, I found myself feeling very impatient waiting with my hand outstretched to have the horse acknowledge me in this way. Again, Lindsey asked me to check in with how I was feeling and share it with her.

"I don't like having to wait for the horse to acknowledge me. I want to just lean in and give her a pat and then rub her ears and neck. I'm not used to needing to be given permission by the horse to touch her," I told Lindsey.

"I can tell you are feeling frustrated by that. Can you see how this transfers to how you are with humans?" she queried.

A bit chagrined, I had to admit, "Yes, I realize that I move right into groups and conversations without getting the social cues of permission." I didn't share this with Lindsey, but I also have developed a bad habit of interrupting someone when they are talking with me or even talking over top of them. It irritates me to no end when I do that, and I'm sure it makes my friends and family even crankier.

Finally, I got the horse handshake from one of the mares, Bella. My third task was assigned. I was to walk in circles around Bella, as close to her body as I felt comfortable. Lindsey and Elisa watched me as I circled Bella from her left flank around her head to her right flank then toward her rump. It was there that I took a wider berth and then moved closer to her body on her left side.

"Okay, what are you feeling?" Elisa asked this time.

"I'm afraid of her hind quarters. I am worried I'm going to be kicked," came my reply. I have been kicked before, so I was wisely cautious of being within reach of Bella's hooves.

Elisa asked me to stop circling and just stand beside Bella.

"Bella is going to give you a sign when and if she feels threatened or gets irritated. I am watching her, and you probably are aware of those signs, too. So far, you can rely on the fact that Bella is predictable and will communicate before kicking," Elisa reassured me, asking me to continue walking slowing around the horse.

I moved around her cautiously, resting my hand on her rump when I circled behind her to reassure myself that she knew I was back there more than anything. Later in future sessions, I was able to trust Bella and rely on her ability to communicate and on my ability to receive her messages.

As of that point, I had only had two sessions with my therapy horse, Bella, in the training arena, and I had already learned so much about myself and how I escalate in communication processes too far, too fast, allowing myself to become stressed. I have also learned that when it comes to getting the horse's attention, my first thoughts and instincts of how to do that involve violence: digging my elbow sharply into her ribs to make her move off the fence rail so I can walk that circle around her.

When Elisa taught me how to ask Bella to move by simply pressing firmly on her side with all ten fingers, I was surprised to feel Bella push back against me, as if to ask, "Are you sure you want me to move?" I then pressed more firmly, as if to say, "Yes, Bella. I want you to move." She pushed back just a little bit longer, and then she moved away. I could definitely see how this communication process transferred into my interactions with humans. I do have the tendency to make more of a scene if what I'm asking for is ignored or there is push-back. This tendency of mine also creates stress in my life!

Another related exercise in the arena helped me understand that I can slowly escalate when I need others to pay attention. I was instructed to get Bella's attention and hold her eye gaze as long as I could in the arena, and I was not to touch her to do so. During this particular session, Bella had given me the green light as soon as I began to approach her, but she just would not give me that horse handshake before we could begin the session. Finally, she quickly sniffed my outstretched hand, and then she dropped her nose again to whiffle around at the weeds in the arena, looking for the specifically tasty ones she wanted to nibble on.

Again, I began to feel frustrated. I almost felt like begging her to look at me, but that didn't feel good, so I didn't do it. Lindsey asked me what other things I might do to draw her attention to me.

"Well, I guess I could clap or jump up and down," I said, half-jokingly.

"Yes! You could wave your arms up and down, jump, clap, or things like that," she agreed with a grin. "Give it a try."

I tried all three of the suggestions she made. Nothing. Bella continued to nibble at the weeds. Elisa came into the center of the arena with three items: a hula hoop, a five-gallon plastic water jug, and a lunge whip. She suggested that I use a prop to capture Bella's attention without touching her. She demonstrated some ways I might use each prop, and then she asked me to choose one and give it a try.

I selected the hula hoop. As I approached Bella, I began to wave the hula hoop up and down then from side to side. I did this several times with no response from my equine partner. Yes, I was frustrated, but I stayed calm, breathing steadily. Finally, Bella looked up from her nibbling and looked straight at me. We stared at each other. It was magical. Then she dropped her head and continued to graze.

"Do it again," Elisa encouraged me. Again? Like that wasn't hard enough? But there must be a reason why I should try again. I felt rather like ending on a high note. Okay. I tried again.

This time, I used the water jug, waving it from side to side and then lifting it up over my head. More quickly this time, Bella stopped grazing and looked at me for a long time. It felt so good! And then Lindsey and I debriefed. We talked about how frustrated I can feel when I need to get someone's attention, and they either ignore my attempts or say they are paying attention but really are distracted by something else. This happens from time to time in my work. And I have not thought about using figurative props; I usually slink away feeling hurt, or I escalate to a higher energetic level than I need to, neither of which is healthy for my strong immune function.

These aha moments in the arena with Bella created a new paradigm for me when it comes to communicating. And a lot has shifted in my company as a result of it. I love equine therapy; I think it will be my therapy technique of choice as I continue to anchor my healing and work on where I can do better with not allowing myself to create the cycles that pull me off center.

Together with this new therapeutic process, learning to live my life with little stress, and learning how to reassure my body that all is well during unavoidable change or stress, I believe I have the tools I need to keep my immune system and digestion functioning at a high level. I understand that times of stress are like times when one might hear an air-raid siren go off. That is the time to go into the bunker and stop doing all of the normal daily tasks. But one cannot live in the bunker. There has to come a time when the all-clear signal sounds, and you can come out and get back to your day-to-day routine. I encourage you to see where this metaphor fits in your own life, and take action before your own health becomes compromised.

BRINGING THE IMMUNE THERAPIES HOME

Beth

I've made many flights home over the years after our international travels to BNI offices all around the world, but thinking back to our flight home from California, after completing my treatment at the Issels Center and having seen Dr. Kelly to learn the tumor was shrinking and the lymph node was normal, is an amazing memory. I think I was emotionally soaring about 60,000 feet above the plane all the way home. I was just so happy that the immune therapies were working. It was clear to us from this scan that my work was paying off.

Next, I had to keep the same level of healing without Dr. Issels and Dr. Kim right there all the time as I implementing Dr. Miller's exhortation to allow no stress into my life for the first six months of my home care. I knew the entire Issels' team was just a phone call away and had sent me home with a good variety of supplements and naturopathic tinctures personally made specifically for me by Dr. Issels to get me started with the nutritional protocol.

I made an appointment right away with my physician's assistant (PA) in Austin to determine which elements of the Issels Protocol I could do at her clinic and what I would need to do elsewhere. I also made an appointment with Dr. Zahir Arifi, an osteopath from France who is practicing in Texas as a massage therapist. I chose to have him do the spinal manipulations that my chiropractor could have done because he also does a lot of soft tissue work and visceral organ manipulation, all of which would support my efforts to optimize my immune system. An added bonus to me is that he uses a quantum biofeedback machine called SCIO to send healing electrical frequencies into my body as needed. SCIO is based on the Rife electrical frequencies that have been used for many years in many countries to weaken cancer cells, so I was very diligent to have this biofeedback scan performed every few weeks during my Healing Bubble time.

One of the first things I did when I sat down with my schedule and the recommendations from the Issels' team was to map out what a month of at-home treatments would look like. I needed to do infrared sauna therapy three times a week, coffee enemas twice a week, hyperbaric chamber three times a week, the autologous cytokines injections every other week, certain IVs every week, others every other week, and still others once a month, along with many new daily disciplines. I have to admit that I was overwhelmed and quite intimidated by having to figure it all out so that I didn't miss anything or do one thing too much and something else not enough.

And then I had a schedule for getting blood tests done. Yikes!

A while before learning about this messenger's presence, I had switched from using a digital, online calendar to creating an artistic bullet journal, or bujo. My bujo makes me so happy! It is brightly colored, and inside are lots of hand-drawn sketches, flourishes, inspirational quotes, and other just generally cute, hand-drawn enhancements to each day's schedule. It helps me with feeling like my life is creative and not just bogged down with tasks. And it makes me metaphorically sing when I open it and plan my time.

I shifted my strategy with my bujo and tracked the at-home treatments in it rather than other kinds of engagements for that first month. I also made a spreadsheet that I taped to my pantry cabinet with the new supplement schedule. Since I would be gone before breakfast and lunch on certain days to have my IVs done at the clinic in Austin and I usually set out Ivan's supplements at the same time as mine, I also made a spreadsheet for Ivan, so he could keep up with his own supplement schedule. I'm not the world's most organized person, but I knew that I needed some sound strategies to keep my regimen on track.

There were a few additional things not specifically prescribed by Dr. Issels that I knew I wanted to do—for example, the equine therapy I mentioned in the previous chapter. I included them in my bujo tracker.

I would have two months to do my at-home therapies before I did another scan. It was more than a little nerve-racking to have to wait two months to know if all the things I was doing were having the powerful, positive impact that I wanted and expected. I was marking the days until I would return to Pasadena, California, to see Dr. Kelly again.

My days began to take on a new rhythm—a new, normal-for-now pattern.

Here's a sample of what a couple of days looked like in my schedule:

- ❖ Monday
  - ➢ Contemplative prayer/meditation
  - ➢ AM Qigong practice
  - ➢ Preparation of supplements for the day
  - ➢ After breakfast, skin brushing
  - ➢ Saltwater soak
  - ➢ Coffee enemas (2)
  - ➢ Check email/Facebook
  - ➢ Lunch
  - ➢ Glutathione IVs at clinic
  - ➢ Hyperbaric chamber treatment at clinic
  - ➢ Supper
  - ➢ Relax with Ivan, watch a couple of TV shows
  - ➢ Retire about 8:30 pm to darkness for night-time routine
  - ➢ Meditation/visualizations
  - ➢ PM Qigong practice

- ➢ Watch funny videos on YouTube and laugh (wearing blue-light blocking glasses)
- ➢ Thymus tapping for ten minutes
- ➢ Asleep by 10 PM

- ❖ Tuesday

  - ➢ Contemplative prayer/meditation
  - ➢ AM Qigong practice
  - ➢ Preparation of supplements for the day
  - ➢ After breakfast, skin brushing
  - ➢ Saltwater soak
  - ➢ Check email/Facebook
  - ➢ Lunch
  - ➢ Hyperthermia treatment
  - ➢ Writing/Relaxing
  - ➢ Supper
  - ➢ Relax with Ivan
  - ➢ Retire about 8:30 pm to darkness for night-time routine
  - ➢ Meditation/visualizations
  - ➢ PM Qigong practice
  - ➢ Watch funny videos on YouTube and laugh (wearing blue-light blocking glasses)
  - ➢ Thymus tapping for ten minutes
  - ➢ Asleep by 10 PM

One of the great joys for me and Ivan in living where we do on Lake Austin is the amount of wildlife we have on and around our property. With the new pattern of my days, I noticed more often what was moving around outside, even though it was so hot in the summer that we rarely poked our noses out the door. We have large windows on the east and west sides of our home and our property on a north-to-south hill, so the deer come onto our property at the top of the hill and meander down to the bottom, and we can watch them from indoors, where it is cool, for hours. That spring, we had quite a crop of fawns, and watching them grow and thrive was a joy.

We also have a pair of wild turkeys that like to hang out around our neighborhood. Sometimes I will walk past my front porch windows and there they will be, lying in our grass taking a nice little nap. It makes me feel so peaceful to see them there. Being in nature, observing wildlife, even listing to the running water of a creek or waterfall are all things that center me and help me regain my peaceful core. These things also up-modulate our immune function.

I was able to put a little garden in, even though by the time I returned to Austin, it was quite late for doing so. Oh, how I love to dig in the dirt! I talk to my plants (Yes, I am a tree hugger. One time my dry-cleaning delivery truck headed down my driveway while I was in full hug with one of my beloved oak trees in front of my house), and I also talk to the little critters that join me in the garden — the lizards, toads, and sometimes, little snakes.

My sweet friend, Kristi, had started seedlings for me while I was away. She brought them over when I had been home a week or two, and we planted them together. Ivan and I enjoyed vine-ripened tomatoes every day for many months to follow.

Being out in my yard in the morning hours and again as the sun sets brings me a lot of joy. As I walked this healing journey, keeping my life simpler was very important. I can still hear Dr. Miller admonishing me, "No stress, Beth. None." And so, I have embraced a gentler, kinder life that is more in tune and in touch with nature and feeds my soul.

I am a firm believer in the power of positive affirmations, so I posted several notes around my home in places where I would see them often. I posted, "I am healed," in several locations. The other affirmation was a message my t'ai chi instructor, Master Samuel Barnes, had sent me via email before I went to Tijuana.

I wrote this note down and kept it near me even in the hospital. It is still on my mirror at home today: "The cellular transformation is vibrant and complete into wholeness and perfection."

My 53rd birthday approached six weeks after I returned home to Austin. I mentioned earlier that Dr. Arifi uses a quantum biofeedback device called SCIO. The week of my birthday in mid-June, Dr. Arifi reported to me that there was no more cancer cellular frequency picked up in my body by SCIO. That was the most exciting news to me. I started to walk around feeling "I am healed" in every cell of my body. It was wonderful. And following on the heels of this positive result was the rapidly approaching follow-up ultrasound I was going to have the first week of July to confirm the progress of my recovery.

During Ivan's prostate-cancer-healing season, Qigong Master Chunyi Lin had suggested that Ivan do a three-day water fast. It wasn't something Ivan did; however, I remembered this suggestion and asked Master Lin if it would be a good idea for me to do one. He agreed that it would be a very good idea. I poked around on the internet for tips on how to succeed with a three-day water fast since I had never done one before. I had fasted for 24 hours many times, but never for three days.

What I learned was astonishing!

Dr. Valter Longo has been doing clinical studies on the effects of fasting, specifically on longevity and healing cancer. His research at the University of Southern California has shown that both the three-day water fast and the five-day fast-mimicking diet have a dramatic positive impact on cancer. So much so that drug companies are scrambling to produce a drug that will induce the fasting effect in the body. But one could just simply fast. So, I checked with Dr. Kim to be sure it was fine for me to do so, and then I fasted. Since I already had a very healthy eating habit, and I was also not using any caffeinated beverages, I did not need to do the normal preparation needed before launching into a fast. Before doing a fast, it is important to check with your healthcare professional to be sure a fast won't harm you, and then prepare yourself for the fast with the guidance of your healthcare professional.

The ability of water-only fasting for at least 72 hours is believed to weaken cancer cells, because these cells are immature cells without the ability to adjust to harsh conditions in the body, and they cannot respond to starvation like our normal cells can. Fasting is believed to be one of the most effective ways to weaken and induce apoptosis in the cancer stem cells.

During my fast, I increased the frequency of my "fever therapy."

Fever therapy such as hyperthermia (the use of an infrared sauna or an infrared sauna blanket) or Colley Vaccines (the introduction of bacterial fragments into the system to trigger high fevers) are both effective ways to weaken and induce apoptosis in cancer cells and are used by many cancer treatment centers and in nearly all the alternative cancer clinics in Germany. Just as fasting does, fevers also create a harsh environment in the body that cancer cells do not tolerate well, while at the same time inducing a strong response from the immune system. Hyperthermia also creates a strong lymphatic flow, which helps our immune systems spring into action. I asked Dr. Kim about changing my routine during my water-only fast to include daily hyperthermia in my Gizmo sauna blanket. He agreed that it would be good for me to do so.

While I was researching the impact of fasting on cancer cells, I started to learn more about sonic healing and the use of focused ultrasound. I found the Focused Ultrasound Foundation and the book, *The Tumor*, written by John Grisham. This whole topic is completely fascinating to me. While I was researching this approach to healing cancer, I also found research done by Fabian Maman, a French composer and bioenergetics healer, and Hélène Grimal, a biologist at the French National Center for Scientific Research in Paris, who performed an experiment with sound energy and cells. Cancer cells take in the sound waves, but because they are immature cells, their membranes cannot release them. Their membranes are a one-way door. As the intensity of the sound energy grows, the cells eventually rupture and die.

The study by Maman and Grimal used a series of low-volume sounds (30-40 decibels) in the scale of C major played on a xylophone. Using nine notes of the scale (C-D-E-F-G-A-B-C-D) over a 14-minute progression, human uterine cancer cells viewed through a microscope ruptured. When the notes were sung by voice, it only took nine minutes to rupture the cancer cells. The results of this study were so exciting for me to learn about. I found a 15-minute YouTube recording of the C-major scale being toned with crystal bowls, but it only had the first seven notes. I got out my keyboard so that I could complete 14-minute cycles with all nine notes.

Then I had a blinding flash of insight: if I also sang these tones loudly as they were being played, couldn't I create more sound vibration that would penetrate my cells even more effectively since they would be originating within my body? And might this be ever so much more effective while I was doing the water-only fast? I started using sound this way to intentionally do even more to weaken the cancer cells in my body, doing it more frequently during my three-day water fast.

Learning from the Focused Ultrasound Foundation that there are treatment centers in Europe and Asia where focused ultrasound is being used to kill cancer cells was also very exciting! I felt like this was my back-up parachute if the immune therapies I was using needed some added oomph. I found a center in Switzerland that does therapeutic focused ultrasound for breast cancer and bookmarked their page on my web browser in case I needed to come back to this modality in the future.

It was at this same time that I asked Master Lin what kind of qigong would be best to support my cancer-healing journey. He recommended his Spring Forest Qigong Five Elements, something I knew about, but had not practiced regularly. He suggested that I begin to practice this set three times a day for half an hour each session during my fast, which I did, downloading his video set from his website, www.springforestqigong.com. He also invited me to come to Minneapolis for a two-week qigong healing retreat. I tucked that invitation away in my mind, wanting to get to the next scan before deciding what to do afterwards.

I also learned Guo Lin Qigong, a walking form of qigong used in China by many cancer patients with amazing results. I started doing the cancer walk all around my house, in and out of the guest bedrooms, down the halls, and through my living room and kitchen during my fast. It's quite a unique way to walk, but it is also very relaxing and incorporates a lot of breathing—oxygenating my whole body.

So my three days' water-only fast also included daily hyperthermia treatments, Spring Forest Qigong's Five Elements, daily sound therapy, and 45 minutes per day of Guo Lin Qigong. This was how I ended my two months of at-home therapy. All of my blood work was looking great: cancer markers were low, white blood cell count was back in the normal range, and my inflammatory markers were lower than they had been in years. The SCIO scan taken near my birthday in June had shown no cancer cellular frequency, but the mass felt unchanged upon palpation. If anything, it felt fuller, itchy, a bit painful, and hot. But I continued walking around thinking, feeling, and saying, "I am healed!"

HEALING CONTINUES

Beth

As the two-month mark approached, I was getting a little bit anxious about the follow-up ultrasound scan I needed. Although my blood work continued to look great (even better than before, with my white blood cell count finally getting in the perfect range), as I mentioned, the tiny messenger seemed like it was getting a little bit bigger. And there were other changes to the mass in my breast that I did not feel so good about. But I concentrated on keeping a positive focus, remembering my SCIO scan results, and I released worry, simply telling myself to remain peaceful and patient until I could get the information I needed about what impact the immune therapies were having.

I thought about scheduling an ultrasound locally, but there were no radiologists in Austin that I could find who would work with me personally like Dr. Kelly had been doing. There was one doctor who my PA thought might be willing, but he said no. His tech would do the scan; he would review it later, and then send the report to my PA. He would not discuss the scan with me. So, I booked a flight back to Pasadena, California. This time Dr. Mohammad went with me to review the findings with Dr. Kelly after the scan was performed.

Dr. Kelly's technician took me back into the exam room and started the scan while Dr. Kelly was finishing up with another patient. The technician started with the lymph node.

"Well, that is normal," she said and moved on to another area.

I lifted my head up off the pillow. "Wait, go back. What?" I questioned her. "Normal? You mean the one that was angiogenic and enlarged before?"

"Yes," she repeated. "It looks normal. See?" She moved the transducer wand back over the node, and there it was in all its glory. Normal size, normal hilum—nice and white, inside the node.

Wow! I was excited now. Things had to be better with the tumor.

Just then Dr. Kelly joined us, and the technician began to take images of the tumor, which was still there. He watched the screen as she moved over the mass, stopping and recording some still images. It definitely looked different this time, but I could not tell if the difference was a good different or not. He was not saying too much.

She went back to the nodes and showed him the now-normal lymph node. "Yes," he said. "That is looking very good."

After the scan was complete, he invited me to join him back in his office. I asked for Dr. Mohammad to join us, too, and Dr. Kelly agreed to have him sit in the evaluation with us.

As the three of us sat together and reviewed the images, Dr. Kelly began to show me a strange, nearly perfect circle that had appeared off the side of the mass near the site of the intra-tumoral injections. He postulated that the intra-tumoral injection had allowed some of the tumor cells to proliferate in that spot but that my body had very efficiently contained them. He pulled up images from the previous scan and showed me how much darker the image of the tumor was now. He explained that the mass was actually slightly larger now, measuring three centimeters, and looked like it may contain more cancer cells within it, which could explain why it was so dark.

Dr. Mohammad asked a few questions, and I pretty much sat quietly.

When we started to look at the lymph node, the difference was amazing. The image from the last scan two months before showed a very faint hilum and an enlarged node. This scan's image was of a normal, white hilum and a normal-sized node. Dr. Kelly said he thought there was still a little bit of a fight going on in that node and showed me a thin, dark edge between one side of the hilum and the side of the node, but he agreed that this was a vast improvement.

He told me again that the primary mass was not going in the right direction and encouraged me to intensify my efforts to heal. "This is not good. It's time to go to Switzerland," he told me.

"Okay, I'm going to Switzerland," I agreed.

Once outside of Dr. Kelly's office, Dr. Mohammad was encouraging and shared with me some ways to intensify my immune therapy, including ways to harness the healing power of sound therapy in a way I had not been doing. I felt encouraged by the recovery of the lymph node, but I was understandably disappointed that the primary tumor seemed to be going in the wrong direction. Everything else was going so well. The improvement in my blood work had been comforting. And to have confirmation that the metastasis was almost certainly reversed made me feel great but also puzzled.

I pondered and wondered about this all the way back home to Austin on the plane. How could it be that the lymph node had cleared, but the primary tumor might have gotten worse? I was really surprised by this finding, to be honest.

I knew that Dr. Kelly would be sending me the report, and he had sent me home with a memory stick that contained the images from that scan. I just could not understand how the tumor could have gotten worse while the metastasis had cleared.

As soon as I got the report in the mail, I scanned and then emailed it to Dr. Kim and Dr. Issels. Dr. Kim called me. He shared with me that both he and Dr. Issels felt like the immune therapies were working. They have seen cancer healing before going exactly like this. They encouraged me not to become worried or scared, to keep using the immune therapies and have another scan in a month or so.

Well.

Hmmmm.

It was then that I opened the envelope with the memory stick in it so I could take a look at the images from the scan. I loaded the images on my computer. And I immediately noticed something that made me catch my breath.

The image from the color Doppler feature: there was no blood flow in the tumor.

Wait. Stop. What?!

No blood flow? No metabolic activity? No angiogenesis? Could that be possible? Could the tumor be dead?

I called Dr. Kim immediately after emailing these images to him. His evaluation of the situation was encouraging. He told me that I was correct to presume that the lack of blood flow to the tumor might well indicate that the tumor had "died." He also told me that when a tumor dies like this, the body sends in fluids with the immune cells, macrophages that are responsible for breaking down the necrotic mass, helping the body to begin to dismantle and absorb the necrotic cells. It would be expected to have a small bump up in the measurement of the mass, and it would look darker on the scan if it were dead tissue or even scar tissue. Only a PET scan would show if there was any remaining inflammation, and he recommended that I do that type of scan in two months' time.

I emailed Dr. Kelly and asked him about what I had noticed on the scan. He confirmed that the lack of blood flow on the scan might indicate that the tumor was dead. He also suggested that I consider having a PET scan to validate that presumption. I knew I could not wait two months to have this scan, so I talked to my PA about requesting the PET scan in about one month. We got it slated for the end of July. Because I then had the sense that the tumor was no longer active, I pulled out the invitation from Master Lin to come to his clinic for a qigong healing retreat. What better way to support my body as it moved slowly back into homeostasis?

Switzerland would have to wait.

GOING DEEPER WITH MEDICAL QIGONG

Beth

I have been a martial artist since the age of 25 when I started to study an American form of karate based on the Shotokan style of martial arts from Okinawa. I never thought that my study of the martial arts would assist me with healing a serious condition like breast cancer, but it did. Continuing to pursue my black belt through the birth of two children, two rounds of adrenal exhaustion, emotional turmoil, and mood instability, I proudly earned my black belt just after I turned 40.

It was after I became a black belt that I began to study the internal martial arts: t'ai chi, baguazhang, and qigong. I have to be honest when I tell you that I did not quite "get it" for many years, but I continued to train, study, and assimilate what my Qigong Master, Samuel Barnes, was teaching me. I've studied with him for over 14 years now.

During these 14 years, I have also had the opportunity to meet and study with Master Chunyi Lin, whom you have met in the pages of this book already. Slowly I began to learn how to emit qi (energy) to have an immediate healing impact on others.

The first time I used medical qigong to help another was when a friend of ours fell while we were hiking one afternoon in a remote area, rolling her ankle badly, and had to be rescued and driven out. Her injury was so bad that she could not walk at all, and her ankle was huge. Back at our lodging, I offered to do a medical qigong session for her injury. She agreed, and I did a basic blockage-opening technique known as sword fingers while she sat with her foot elevated and iced. We were on a remote island in the British Virgin Islands, and there was no medical facility there to help with her injury. Later that evening, she showed up at the festivities wearing high heels with no swelling of the ankle and no pain. She was completely fine!

The next day, one of the men in our group who was learning how to kite surf was picked up by the wind and slammed forcefully to the ocean. From the height he fell, the surface of the water felt more like cement than water. When he returned to the island, he told us that he had broken ribs before, and he felt that he had broken two or maybe three ribs in this incident.

Not wanting to overstep my very new friendship with him, I asked his partner if it might be acceptable for me to offer to do a medical qigong session with him. The rest of the guests were preparing for a tennis tournament, and he had been planning to play. The pain was so intense that there was no way he was going to play. His partner asked me what it would entail, and I explained the process. They both agreed that I could perform the sword fingers technique with him, and so I did. The session took about three minutes. He got up, stretched gingerly, looked at me with surprise, and then smiled, picked up his tennis racket, and joined the tournament—he was pain free. And he remained pain free until the next morning when he asked for another session before leaving the island to pilot his private plane back to the United States.

Since those first experiences in using medical qigong to benefit others, I have been able to assist more people who have been in excruciating pain, including a young child who was having an IV at the same clinic I was at in Austin for one of my healing infusions. When he arrived with his father and sister, I was sleeping. When his infusion started, he began to really cry. The pain was unbearable for him, poor little guy. I started to surface from my nap, realizing that someone near me was crying. When I woke up fully and realized it was this young child, I asked the nurse if I could offer to do medical qigong to help him with the pain. She agreed, if his father would give his permission, so I explained a bit about medical qigong and what I would be doing.

Both the boy and his father agreed that I could proceed. Within about one minute, the pain started to lift for the child and completely vanished. He finished the infusion with no more pain. As a matter of fact, all his future weekly infusions went well, with no pain. We were getting treatments on the same day, so I was there for him in case he needed me. Gratefully, the one session was all it took.

I tell you these experiences to provide context for my own use of medical qigong to help heal my tumor. Prior to my developing breast cancer, Master Lin had done several medical qigong healing sessions with both me and with Ivan. As a matter of fact, when I first detected the tumor, I called Master Lin, who conducted a medical qigong session with me by phone. I had several more phone sessions with him before I went to Minnesota for the healing retreat.

I set aside ten days to spend in Minnesota—instead of two weeks—because I just did not want to be away from my home again for a long time. Arriving on a Tuesday evening, I drove to place in the country where one of our good friends, Pete, lives. He lives in an earth-sheltered house on eleven wonderfully wooded and landscaped acres. The environment at Pete's is so healing and peaceful. I had the most beautiful vistas and enjoyed his labyrinth made with huge carved stone frogs from Bali called the Frogyrinth. Pete did not mind that I disappeared to the guest quarters around sunset and got up before sunrise. He made me green drinks every morning, and we cooked together in the evening when I returned from the Spring Forest Qigong Center in Eden Prairie. Master Lin graciously invited me to stay with him in his lakefront home for the second half of my retreat.

While I was in Minnesota, I went to the Spring Forest Qigong Center every day. My healing time was quite enjoyable. I was able to work with all three of the master healers at the center. They worked with me in guided meditation, group classes, and seated meditation. I received private medical qigong treatments, practiced the Spring Forest moving qigong, and received qi-ssage, a special form of massage for the purpose of opening energy channels in the body. I spent between five and eight hours per day in qigong practice.

While I stayed with Master Lin, he cooked meals for me with special herbs and mushrooms to support my immune system. He gave me goji berries, red dates, and powdered mushroom blends with reishi mushrooms. We practiced the Spring Forest Qigong Five Elements together in the early morning hours while the lake was waking up. It was wonderful. In the evenings, when he returned from the center, he did additional qi-ssage and qigong healing sessions with me. His focus was to be sure all my energy blockages were opened and that energy was flowing freely in my whole body. He told me that my kidney qi was weak, and he tonified the kidney qi energy. I began to learn a whole new vocabulary for healing and experienced more of the traditional Chinese medicine (TCM) approach to disease and healing. I liked what I was learning.

And the tumor just continued to become smaller and softer, noticeably changing under my skin. I began to feel a deeper level of peacefulness, tranquility, and contentment. Happiness and joy permeated my heart and soul. I smiled even more than I had already been smiling prior to my retreat. The smile lines deepened around my eyes, which I appreciated.

During my earlier research into qigong healing and cancer, I had come across a video of a patient with a bladder tumor, who was treated at a medicine-less qigong hospital in China. On video you can watch the qigong masters working on the patient while the patient's bladder tumor is being scanned and is clearly visible on the monitor beside her. As the medical qigong treatment progresses, the tumor seems to quickly shrink and then completely disappear.

I asked Master Lin about this video, specifically whether or not it was valid. He knew of the case, and he said it was verified. I asked him what the qigong masters were chanting during the treatment. He told me that they were saying, "Already healed" in Chinese. A large part of the healing realized with qigong involves feeling healed, knowing you are healed, and then you become healed, because the body is malleable by the mind.

I tucked this bit of information into my memory.

Then Master Lin told me that the patient had later died from a recurrence of the cancer. In his opinion it was because the focus had been exclusively on the tumor and not on removing the energy blockages in the whole body and tonifying the qi.

Traditional Chinese medicine's approach to illness is that disease arises when there is an imbalance in yin and yang energies, blockages in energy channels, and weakness in qi in the body. This has been a new way for me to look at illness, especially cancer. And I have very much enjoyed learning and applying the principles of qigong to my recovery.

According to the principles of qigong, I had a blockage in the lung channels compounded by weak kidney qi which supports healthy lung qi. Blockages in the lung channels can lead to congestion, cysts, and tumors, both malignant and benign, in the breasts. I do have a history of cysts, and I did ultimately develop a malignant tumor.

I practiced qigong healing exercises to open the blockage in my lung channels, and I also did a lot of qigong to balance the yin and yang energy in my entire body, as well as tonify and purify my qi. When I was at Master Lin's clinic in Minnesota, he confirmed that I had too much yang energy and not enough yin energy. Yang energy is the doing energy; yin energy is the being energy. There was no doubt that I was doing more than being for quite a few years leading up to the detection of this tiny messenger.

Later, upon my return home from the Spring Forest Qigong Center, I got online and ordered Dr. Jerry Alan Johnson's five-volume *The Secret Teachings of Chinese Energetic Medicine*. I also visited our local Asian market and brought home a variety of mushrooms, organic sprouted grains, goji berries, and red dates. I wanted to continue what I had been doing at Master Lin's once I was at home. I also did a search for a local TCM practitioner in Austin. I found Dr. Nelson Song Luo, a faculty member at the AOMA Graduate School for Integrative Medicine, and made an appointment with him to continue having my qi balanced and strengthened. I chose Dr. Luo because he had a deep understanding of qigong and TCM.

Dr. Luo started working with my qi, my life energy. He commented right away that my kidney qi was too weak. He did acupuncture using many points during a single treatment. He noticed that my hearing is not as good as it could be and that I have a lot of tinnitus, both manifestations of weak kidney qi.

He did "hot needling" with moxa sticks (I liked that a lot) and some electric stimulation to my ears. As I learned more about the kidney channel and its connection to the ears, I realized that my body had been telling me for a long time that my kidney qi was getting too weak. I simply did not understand the signs the body had been using to let me know this.

My second visit to Dr. Luo found my kidney qi to still be strong from my first treatment and the qigong healing work I was doing at home. My subsequent experience is that my kidney qi continues to be strong with most of the visits I have had, only dipping after travel.

Dr. Luo also prescribed a variety of dried herbs to "cool heat" and "dry dampness." The way TCM approaches the body is very different from our allopathic (modern Western medicine) approach. Where we might refer to inflammation, TCM refers to heat. Where we talk about stress and anxiety, TCM talks about too much yang energy or an imbalance in yin and yang energies.

There is no doubt in my own mind that my experience with cancer resulted from too much yang energy in my life, too much activity, too much thinking, doing, and worrying, and not enough relaxing, resting, centering in, and breathing.

Every day I went to the Spring Forest Qigong Center in Minnesota, the healers and I could feel that my qi was getting stronger and more balanced. One day I felt an ant crawling through the hairs on my right forearm during one of the healing sessions. My eyes were closed, and I was totally relaxed. I did not want to come out of my relaxed state to look down to brush the ant off my arm. But it kept crawling and tickling my arm. I reluctantly opened one eye just a tiny bit to glance down at the ant because by then, it was distracting me too much. There was nothing there!

I looked up in surprise at the qigong practitioner who was smiling at me.

"Did you feel that?" she asked me.

"Yes, I thought there was an ant crawling on my arm," I replied in disbelief.

"I felt it too, on my arm. The lung energy channel is opening up," she reassured me.

I closed my eyes and went back into my deep relaxation.

On the last day that I was with the qigong practitioners, the same qigong healer was working with me toward the end of the day. As I sat there quietly, breathing deeply, slowly, and relaxing, I suddenly started to feel a tingling sensation in the area of the tumor. It was a bit like static electricity, not painful, but not like anything I had ever felt before. Again, I partially cracked open one eye to see what was happening around me. The practitioner was calmly reaching into the air in front of me and pulling something away repeatedly.

"What is it?" I asked.

"There was a beautiful orchid in your breast. I removed it." She smiled peacefully at me. I smiled back at her, thought to myself, *already healed,* and closed my eyes with deep joy and contentment.

Millions of people in the world rely on medical qigong for their healthcare, and they heal gently, easily, and gracefully. Why couldn't this form of healing work for me? Of course, it could! Master Lin has many students who have their cancers reverse completely and who go on to live a full life when they follow his instruction to keep their lives balanced and centered on the most powerful healing energy in the entire universe: unconditional love.

I believe the reason I healed as quickly as I did was because I used medical qigong along with all that was available to me from Western medicine's understanding of non-toxic, natural therapies that worked in harmony with my body's innate healing capacity, not against it. And while medical qigong is not something that most of us know anything about, TCM is growing in our country as a viable way to seek treatment for illness alongside other strategies. Finding a TCM practitioner who can work together with your naturopathic doctor or your integrative medical doctor will serve you well in your own healing journey. More and more alternative healthcare clinics are including some aspect of TCM, as allopathic practitioners come to more highly respect and trust this approach to health. Even high-tech oncology centers are using some aspects of TCM, usually acupuncture and t'ai chi/qigong, to support their patients.

Using qigong in my healing journey has so profoundly impacted me that I have entered into a three-year medical qigong practitioner program. It is one more way I can help others experience the abundant health I know is waiting for them.

HEALING IS COMPLETE

Beth

While I spent the month of July focused on working with my energy in this gentle, internal way, the mass continued to get smaller and smaller. I did all I could to support this part of my healing process. I stayed hydrated, rested a lot, slept about eleven hours per night, and nourished my body with highly nutritious foods.

I also started to work more closely with my good friend, Dr. Lise Janelle, and experiencing her Heart Freedom Method. The Heart Freedom Method took me deeper into the BodyMind, finding that one of the conclusions formed by my subconscious mind when I was unable to understand things happening around me was that "it is not good for others that I was alive." I found it very interesting that this subconscious programming had guided my body into a condition that had the potential to kill me. We started working together regularly, and Dr. Lise began teaching me her method so I can use it to work with my own Abundant Health clients. She was able to gently reteach my subconscious about the conclusion it had formed, and it helped my conscious and my subconscious work together toward my healing even more quickly. I cannot stress how important it is to have ALL of your mind in agreement about your healing process. This is probably one of the least understood and least implemented protocols when it comes to physical healing. Our minds are the most important tools for healing that we possess. The Heart Freedom Method helped me be sure all of my mind was focused on healing.

So now the end of July was quickly approaching, and it was time to book my PET scan. With great anticipation, I made the appointment and trotted off to have my scan. Oh, how I tried to get the technician to share any little tiny hint about what she saw on the screen while performing the scan, but she would have none of it. So, I patiently waited for the report to be sent to my doctor (*not!*).

This time, when the report came in, the PA would not allow it to be sent to me until after she reviewed it. My PA was not going to be in the office for a week, and she did not want me to simply receive the report without being able to hear what the values meant and what it seemed to be revealing, so her nurse sent the report directly to Dr. Kim, who called me to go over it with me.

The PET scan was inconclusive. Sheesh. This was the test that was supposed to be able to verify with certainty whether or not the tumor was finally dead. What it did verify was that it had decreased in size by over 50%, going from 3 cm to 1.4 cm in that short month! There were quite a few areas showing inflammation but not conclusive for malignancy. Dr. Kim explained to me, once again, that this was what they normally expected to see if my lymphatic system were absorbing the necrotic tissue and breaking it down. There was a small amount of inflammation in the primary tumor, with lower levels of inflammation in several lymph nodes.

There were also three very small spots of inflammation on the outer lining of my right lung. While not conclusive for spread of cancer, it still caught Dr. Kim's attention. There was no way to know, he told me, if the current levels of inflammation represented interval improvement or something new. He asked me to consider starting two medications to stop estrogen production in my body because two out of three breast cancers are estrogen dominant. If the cancer cells my body had developed were fueled by estrogen, then taking the medications would help to reduce the available energy for any remaining malignant cells. That made sense to me, so I agreed. One of these medications was Arimidex, an aromatase inhibitor.

He also suggested that I start a targeted cytotoxic oral therapy at a very low dose. Here, I balked. In my mind, this PET scan was a win: no high levels of inflammation, but rather the levels of inflammation to be expected if the tumor were being broken down, as it clearly was, having shrunken from 3 cm to 1.4 cm. I was not worried in the least about inflammation on the outer lining of my lung. But I had to admit that the low dose chemotherapy he was recommending would be best taken now if these three spots were, in fact, malignant spots which were growing. But again, I really did not want to do treatments that suppress my immune system, working against the normal processes of the body.

Dr. Kim explained to me that the low dose he was recommending would be expected to have no deleterious effects on my body. It should not suppress my immune system or even cause me to feel nauseated. He told me he has seen a 99% rate of success with tumors resolving very quickly with a two-week course of the medication, called Xeloda.

I discussed this at length with Ivan and a couple of my other doctors, and none of them felt like it would be the wrong thing to do. After sitting with the idea for a few days myself, I agreed to do it, even though I felt to my core that it was not necessary. But better to not zig when I should have zagged, I thought.

Getting the medications was not as easy as you might think it would be. Up until that point, most of what I had been doing to heal cancer naturally was not been covered by my insurance. Then, when I needed to use my medical insurance, suddenly I had to jump through a lot of hoops. And I learned just how expensive traditional cancer treatments are! One of the medications was a shot I would need once a month before I could even start on Arimidex. It cost $1,500 per injection, and I needed to have three of them. And the oral chemotherapy, Xeloda, cost $4,500 for the typical three-week prescription of four tablets per day! Although I was only going to take one tablet per day for two weeks (14 tablets), I could only receive the full course of 84 tablets. There was no option for my insurance to pay for the lower number of tablets. They would only authorize payment on the full course.

It was during this part of my healing journey that I learned the FDA had just approved an immunotherapy for clinical trials similar to what the Issels ImmunoOncology Hospital had done for me in Mexico, with the twist that instead of simply activating the patients' immune cells, the lymphocytes are genetically modified (and thus patented) and then put back into the patients' bodies. This process causes a reaction in some patients, who then need two other medications to keep the body's immune system from going so haywire that it actually kills the patient. This type of chemical immunotherapy costs $475,000! My entire treatment at Issels was under one-fifth of this amount. It feels wrong that insurance will pay so much money for drugs that are quite toxic and have serious side effects, even resulting in the patient's death, but they will not pay for treatments that are natural, non-toxic, and effective.

I had gotten a little taste of the standard-of-care cancer machine when I went to the surgeon at MD Anderson in Houston, Texas. Now I was learning more about the extreme pharmaceutical expenses relating to cancer treatment. We seem to turn a blind eye as consumers to these costs because our insurance will cover them. But now our insurance premiums are getting higher and higher, until many people cannot even afford to carry insurance anymore, and we wonder why.

The aromatase inhibiter was approved by my pharmaceutical coverage on my current insurance plan, but the shots I needed to have first in order to take it was not. Really? The injections of Lupron needed to be billed to the medical side of my insurance plan, rather than the pharmaceutical side, so I had even more hoops to jump through. I finally received word from my insurance that they would approve payment of the drugs being prescribed for me.

Xeloda and Lupron are considered specialty medications and needed to be ordered from a specialty pharmacy. I was about to be introduced to yet another machine. After making several calls to arrange the delivery of these medications, a large package arrived via FedEx. Inside the package was a branded cooler containing the meds with a branded tote bag, a wipe-off calendar with the company logo and dry erase marker, as well as a blank journal (also marked with the logo) in which to take note of any side effects to discuss with my doctor. I can tell you that I have never received gifts before from any other pharmacies.

Shortly after starting the targeted oral therapy, the immunologist in Mexico invited me to come back to have another round of non-toxic immunotherapy to support my healing process, just in case the lung lesions were something undesirable trying to get started. I felt much more on board with doing more immunotherapy, rather than using chemotherapy. So, after consulting with Dr. Kim, who agreed with the immunologist, I discontinued Xeloda after only 11 days, because I needed to have it out of my system before returning to the Issels ImmunoOncology Hospital. Those were the most expensive 11 pills I have ever taken, and I felt completely disoriented by taking chemo at all. I was only too happy to stop that course of treatment. I reasoned with Dr. Kim that if the immunotherapy did not seem to work for me the second time, I could resume the cyto-toxic, targeted therapy. Dr. Kim and I agreed that I would continue taking Arimidex, the aromatase inhibitor, to keep my estrogen levels as low as possible, again, "just in case" the lung lesions were metastatic tumors containing estrogen-dominant breast cancer cells.

After the targeted oral therapy, from which I had no side effects whatsoever, Ivan and I returned to the Issels ImmunoOncology Hospital for what ended up being my final round of cancer vaccines. This time they sent a driver to our hotel in San Diego to bring us to the hospital where I had blood drawn so my vaccine could be made. It was wonderful to see my doctors there who joined me in celebrating the great results achieved thus far along my healing journey.

Since it did not take as long to prepare the booster vaccination, there was no need for me to stay in the hospital receiving other treatments. I returned to San Diego immediately after having the blood drawn to make the vaccines. Two days later, we were again driven into Mexico in order for me to receive the activated LAK and NK cells that had been prepared for me. I was so excited to see the IV bag with my activated cells in it. The bag needed to be warmed, so I gratefully held it between my palms, then pressed it against my heart, sending in love, gratitude, and joy to the cells waiting to rejoin the rest of my immune system's cells. The nurse started the IV so that the life-giving cells could be infused into my bloodstream. Since all that was left of the tumor was the small bit of scar tissue which was seen in the ultrasound and PET scan performed at the end of July, there was no need to do an intra-tumoral injection, so that part of the treatment was not repeated.

Both Ivan and I were surprised at how quickly the infusion went. Just like the first time, I started to get a scratchy, then sore, throat. My back began to ache, and by the time we left the laboratory, I had a low-grade fever. I had this low fever for about six hours. My immune response was again triggered. I had wondered if I would have the same response, given that the primary tumor was no longer metabolically active, and the lymph node was normal—signs that there would be fewer cancer cells for my immune system to react to. When I asked the immunologist about this, she assured me that I should experience just as strong a response since the reaction was based on how aggressive the incoming cells were, not on how much there was in the body to react to. Well, this much was for certain, I had a strong immune response!

Once the infusion was complete, we were driven back into California straight to the airport for our return flight home to Texas. I think I had the biggest, widest smile on my face the entire flight home. My heart was feeling so light, and I was completely elated, confident that my own cells were going to accomplish the final "clean-up" of any remaining cancer cells in my body. Not long after my return home, the immunologist emailed me the report of CTCs (circulating tumor cells) in this recent sample: zero.

After learning that my CTC count was zero, both Dr. Kim and Dr. Issels congratulated me and encouraged me to make no changes to my at-home care. They wanted me to pass the six-month point from the original immunotherapy and to then continue with the same at-home treatments for one more month in order to anchor this marvelous healing. And they did want me to do one final high-definition, color Doppler ultrasound to verify that the tumor was breaking up and being absorbed.

It was during this seventh month of my entire treatment protocol that the aromatase inhibitor (AI) began to cause pain in my body. Virtually all of the patients who use this class of medications experience joint and muscle pain, and I was no different. I knew in advance this might be a side effect that would show up. Long-term use can actually cause arthritis and other debilitating conditions. After receiving the CTC count of zero and consulting with Dr. Kim, I discontinued Arimidex one month early and slowly began to have fewer aches and pains. I did some personal research into natural aromatase inhibitors and learned that grapeseed extract, cabernet sauvignon, mangosteen rind, and miso have been clinically studied as strong, natural AIs in a study undertaken by the National Institute of Health. Since I had received a zero CTC count, I did not focus on these natural aromatase inhibitors, although I did begin to use a supplement called DIM to keep my estrogen balanced, not allowing estrone to become elevated, as it had been prior to my diagnosis.

I also learned that pharmaceutical AIs were not subjected to long-term studies before they were approved for patient use by the FDA. This alarms me, and it should alarm you, too! Research doctors and the pharmaceutical companies just do not know what the deleterious long-term impacts of this class of drugs are. And there is no evidence that they have a stronger effect on estrogen-dominant breast cancers than Tamoxifen, which also can have debilitating side effects. Most women with hormone-dependent breast cancer are put on Tamoxifen first for five to ten years, and then they are moved on to aromatase inhibitors such as Arimidex for another five to ten years. I felt comfortable using what Dr. Kim had recommended, and he felt comfortable with my decision ultimately to discontinue the AI, given the additional information we received about the positive direction my condition was going. This is a perfect example of what Ivan and I mean when we say that you must be the captain of your own ship and find a doctor who will work with you and not bully you into something about which you feel great resistance. In the heat of the moment, don't let your doctor bully you with fear or push you into something you do not feel good about. Our recommendation is that you tell them you will take it under advisement, then step away, and breathe. Get more information and consult some other well-informed healthcare professionals, so you have a complete picture of your options. Your doctors work for you. If they browbeat you, fire them.

What I would learn next confirmed that discontinuing the medication at this point was not going to be a problem at all for me.

Prior to a convention that our company, BNI, was holding in Long Beach, California, I booked another ultrasound with Dr. Kelly in nearby Pasadena. By now it had been a little over three months after my booster vaccine in Mexico. This time Dr. Chan, a visiting physician, was with Dr. Kelly to be trained on use of the automated breast ultrasound technology because he was interested in taking the SonoCine machines to China for early breast cancer detection. Dr. Chan is an associate professor from USC who had been studying breast cancer for 18 years. With my okay, he was invited to sit in on my scan and the subsequent report.

Dr. Kelly was aware that my PET scan had shown that the tumor had rapidly shrunk. He was very interested to see how the tumor was doing. As the scan started, Dr. Kelly explained to Dr. Chan that the tumor had been so large that it was easily visible under the skin, and now there was nothing to see. He told Dr. Chan about the lymph node and moved the transducer over the right axillary area to show him the now completely normal lymph node.

And then he moved the transducer over the remains of the tumor.

"Look at that!" Dr. Kelly exclaimed. He pointed to the monitor. Dr. Chan knew the significance of what Dr. Kelly was pointing out, but I did not. I could still see the outline of the tumor, but it did not seem as dark. I did not notice that the mass was no longer spiky like that Tim Burton Christmas tree.

After concluding the scan, the doctors went into the office, and I dressed and joined them. We looked at my scan from July and compared it to this scan. It was clearly different. The tumor was both smaller and smoother, and healthy tissue was filling it in. It now measured 1.2 cm.

"This is irrefutable," Dr. Kelly told us. "The tumor is dead, and it is breaking up."

He showed us the color Doppler image, which showed no angiogenesis in the tumor. He explained what this meant to Dr. Chan, who also seemed extremely pleased with my result. Being a TCM practitioner before coming to the United States, Dr. Chan was fascinated by the fact I had used the healing practices of qigong and acupuncture during my healing journey.

Before I left Dr. Kelly's office, I asked him what he thought about repeating the PET scan now to verify that the lung lesions had resolved. After asking me a series of questions about my inflammatory markers from my blood work, which were all still low, and hearing that my CTC count was zero, he counseled me not to worry about the lesions at this time. It would not be beneficial to subject my body to the additional radiation to repeat the PET scan. His recommendation was to consider repeating that scan in a year's time, November 2018. This seemed like wise counsel to me. I ran this by Dr. Kim afterwards, who agreed with Dr. Kelly.

I left Dr. Kelly's office filled with joy, filled with peace, and filled with celebration. It was over. The transition of the tumor to normal tissue over the previous nine months was irrefutable. I had completely healed.

Was this healing process complicated?

You bet!

It took so much dedication, understanding, research, reading, questioning, learning, focus, and courage, but it happened easily and quickly. My body wanted to heal. Using the BodyMind was a powerful way to approach healing. And I'm not the only one who has had this experience.

I believed from the very beginning that there is a better and safer way to heal cancer, and now I know for sure that there is! I also understand now from personal experience that it takes a lot of courage to live with cancer while doing everything possible to optimize the immune system and weaken cancer cells in order for the body to slowly correct the imbalances that have developed and return the body to health. It can seem so much more of a sure "cure" to work with your oncologist to remove the malignant mass(es) or use the strongest poison possible to shrink tumors as quickly as possible, so they can be surgically removed as soon as possible. The problem is that the systemic cause of the imbalance that suppressed the immune system and allowed the cancer to proliferate unchecked is never addressed with that approach.

Most of us know and accept that the tests typically used to screen and diagnose cancer are carcinogenic. Yet, there are non-carcinogenic screening processes, like automated breast ultrasound, able to detect smaller cancers sooner, but most doctors do not recommend this screening technique, preferring instead to send women to have yearly (or even more often) mammograms, which are known to expose us to cancer-causing X-rays.

Many cancer patients have no understanding of what got them to a cancer diagnosis in the first place. Worse yet, they are actually told by their oncologists that what they eat will have no impact on their condition—"keep eating whatever you want, whatever you can get in your body." The patients may believe that they were simply genetically predisposed for cancer or that some environmental cause led to their diagnoses. While this may be true, I believe that the answer for many, many cancer patients can be optimizing the immune system and enacting many different, natural approaches that weaken cancer cells. I also believe the research on epigenetics reveals that we do not always develop the conditions our genetics seem to indicate are our destiny.

I am not the only person in the world to have had this kind of gentle and rapid result with the approach I took to healing cancer. And as more people like my husband and me share our experiences, we believe the more commonplace a non-toxic, natural approach will become—it is possible to gently, quickly, and easily heal cancer! When I studied the metadata about all cancers and all types of chemotherapy and learned it is a small percentage of cases in which chemotherapy actually works to resolve the primary tumor and/or no secondary tumors form, my choice seemed more logical and sensible than getting caught up in the cancer treatment machine that has become the standard of care. I have seen too many studies about the return of cancers in the majority of people who select the standard of care as their treatment, often due to the carcinogenic nature of the treatments themselves: chemotherapy and radiation, not to mention more frequent scans to monitor the patients' conditions, exposing them to even more carcinogenic radiation.

And then there are the people who go into spontaneous remission for no apparent, explainable reason. Why couldn't that be my own reality, too? I choose to believe that it could have been.

While every reader won't agree with me and may not choose integrative medicine for healing cancer, I know there will be some who want to believe it can work. I hope my story will be reassuring to you that there is another way!

PART TWO:
EDUCATIONAL CONTENT

I Remembered

By Beth Misner

When I was told I had breast cancer,
I remembered a lot of things.

I remembered I used to sing.
I remembered I used to write music.
I used to dance; I used to compose poetry.
I remembered a lot of things.

When did I forget these things?
And why?

In my heart, I knew my complete recovery
Was centered on remembering.

The following section highlights key elements of the Misner Plan's method for boosting immune function and weakening cancer cells in addition to the dietary aspect of the plan, which is covered in detail in our previous book, *Healing Begins in the Kitchen*.

If you have recently been told you are on a similar cancer healing journey to what we have been on, you may already be feeling overwhelmed and at a loss for where to start making changes. We hope Beth's story has brought you hope and encouragement that a non-toxic, integrative approach to restoring health can help your body recover completely. The first chapter in this section will address where to start.

To support you in your own experience, we recommend that you approach our educational content this way: First, read through the two summary chapters and the elaboration that follows, and then begin looking for a healthcare practitioner who can help you captain your ship, using aspects of the Misner Plan that may be appropriate for you. After that, educate yourself further with the recommended reading we list in the resource section at the end of this book.

This book is not meant to be instructional for your specific condition. Beth and Ivan are not medical doctors. While Betty Runkle holds a doctorate in traditional naturopathy, she is not your personal healthcare provider, and her suggestions are made here as information only, not as an attempt to diagnose or prescribe treatment for you. We don't know what the current state of your body's toxic burden is or what other issues you may be dealing with that we did not have to address, such as parasitic infestation or other co-morbid health conditions such as high blood pressure, diabetes, or heart disease.

You will want to have an integrative medical doctor, naturopath, or traditional Chinese medicine (TCM) doctor work specifically with you. They will approach your healing path in a non-toxic, natural way that focuses more on your whole body system and not exclusively on the evidence for a systemic breakdown in your body: malignancy.

We have provided some referrals in the back of the book to healthcare providers in the United States, Mexico, and Germany that the Misner Plan stands behind and recommends. If you would like some more specific referrals in your area to alternative healthcare practitioners, please contact us through our website: www.MisnerPlan.com.

DIAGNOSED WITH CANCER–
WHAT TO DO FIRST

Ivan and Beth

Words from our doctors have so much power: "This is cancer." Instantly, most of us feel fear wash over us, almost ripping through our brains like a lightning bolt, streaming down through our tissues, and lodging as a pit in the bottoms of the stomach or a lump in the throat. We have been conditioned in our society to fear cancer and the intense, painful, and debilitating road that conventional cancer treatment is for most people who experience it. We all know many people, some who are closest to us, who have died horrible, painful deaths from cancer and the side effects of the current medical standard of care to treat cancer. And our Western doctors, doctors trained in allopathic medicine, with their approach of diagnosing and treating symptoms with drugs, radiation, and surgery, have no other paradigm from which to approach cancer. They are frightened for us!

But this is not how large numbers of medical doctors in other countries react to a cancer diagnosis. And it is not how those doctors who are trained in the systemic care of the body using non-toxic, natural therapies respond, either.

The United States is not the only country in which it is illegal for a medical doctor to treat cancer with alternative healthcare. The United Kingdom is perhaps even more punitive with their doctors who stray from the established standard of care than the United States is. Our good friends, Brian and Lynne McTaggart, are doing great work to share hope in the UK with their publication, *What Doctors*

Don't Tell You, in which science-based outcomes of the research studies on non-toxic cancer treatments are shared.

There is a different way.

If you are looking for a different way, we're so glad you have read Beth's story, and we encourage you to read Ivan's story in *Healing Begins in the Kitchen.* We know from experience that you are asking, "What do I do first?"

Let's start from the beginning: you have a suspicious lump or a blood test result that seems to indicate cancer. Medical doctors are going to usually go straight to ordering a biopsy to check the tissue and the pathology of the cells. But as you read in Beth's story, they are not able to tell you that there are no risks to tissue biopsies. The risks range from infection to tracking, which can seed new tumors elsewhere in your body. We did not know this when Ivan was first told, "You need a biopsy."

Blood biopsies are being pursued more often in our country because of the risks associated with repeat biopsies. But we would like to know about the risks associated with the primary biopsy; when can we rely on our medical professionals to protect us from these risks, too?

This is why we requested that our doctors perform additional imaging and other diagnostic procedures to get the information we needed in order to make the choices we wanted to make regarding our healing process.

When Ivan seemingly came out of remission, he knew that surgery or radiation was not the path he wanted to go down. He had healed once, and he wanted to give his body the chance to heal again. Without a biopsy. And, boy, did his urologist sputter and fume over that, but gratefully, he was willing to follow Ivan's progress by ordering MRI and ultrasound scans. When the scans showed progress toward healing, he stopped pressuring Ivan to do a repeat biopsy.

When my (Beth's) MD Anderson oncologist wanted me to have four biopsies, I firmly replied, "No, thank you." I knew there were other diagnostic tests that could evaluate how likely it was that my tiny messenger was malignant. And although my understanding of the body as a system in which cancer was arising as a symptom was not as clear then as it would later become, I knew also that chemotherapy, surgery, and radiation were not the path toward healing for me. I would later learn that there are many doctors practicing medicine today around the whole world who don't need to know much about the cellular composition of the tumor to actually boost immune function, weaken those damaged cells, and induce the healing response in the body. It did not matter whether my tumor was ER+, PR+, or HER2. We did not need to know the precise cellular pathology in order for me to gently and thoroughly return to complete health.

Although Ivan did have a tissue biopsy when prostate cancer was first suspected by his urologist in 2012, none of the subsequent diagnostic scans he had, nor the diagnostic scans I had, are considered capable of returning a confirmed cancer diagnosis in the United States. As we went through our respective healing journeys, we learned the ranking system assigned to prostate scans (Pi-Rads) and breast scans (Bi-Rads) can only give a staged percentage of likelihood that a subsequent biopsy would return a positive diagnosis. The lower the score, the less likely the lesion or tumor in question will be malignant. About 3-5% of Bi-Rads 5, the highest score given before confirmation of breast cancer by biopsy (and the score all my diagnostic scans returned), are actually not malignant, according to peer-reviewed studies published by the Radiological Society of North America and the American College of Radiology.

Here are some of the least carcinogenic scans and tests you can ask for:

- High definition, color Doppler ultrasound (The color Doppler function will show if the mass has a source of blood flow.)

- Automated Breast Ultrasound or SonoCine

- 3T MRI with and without contrast (This will show if there is poor cell differentiation, typical in malignant masses.)

Here are some blood tests you can ask for:

- OncoStat Plus blood test by the Research Genetic Cancer Center (RGCC) in Greece

- ONCOblot blood test (ENOX2 protein test) available in limited availability but coming fully to United States' patients soon

- Nagalese blood levels (Nagalese is a protein that cancer cells produce.)

In addition, a PET scan can evaluate high levels of inflammation and may show where other malignant lesions may have metastasized. It is important to know that a PET scan measures inflammation, and if your body is breaking down a "dead" tumor in the breast, there is going to naturally be more inflammation in the lymph nodes near the tumor as the body uses white blood cells to carry cellular debris into the lymph in order to move it out of the body through the kidneys and ultimately the bladder.

When my tumor was less than half its size at the largest measurement, there were actually eight lymph nodes with low levels of inflammation seen in my PET scan. It took the skilled eye of an experienced nuclear radiologist to recognize that this was exactly what would be expected while my body was dismantling the necrotic tissue.

Remember that PET scans expose the body to quite a high level of carcinogenic radiation—the equivalent of about 50 chest X-rays, so you may wish for your practitioner to evaluate if and when you should have PET scans, depending on your condition. It was recommended to me that I not repeat this diagnostic test for at least a year after the first one if ultrasounds and blood work were all continuing to show stability. The risks to my body outweighed the benefits of the information this type of scan would give my medical team.

Some immuno-oncology centers in Mexico, like the Issels ImmunoOncology Hospital, will isolate, count, and phenotype cancer cells, circulating tumor cells, and circulating (malignant) stem cells. While this is not considered technically to be a blood biopsy, it does provide certainty that a highly suspicious lesion is malignant. If there is no malignant tumor, there will be no malignant tumor cells being released into your blood stream.

Once you have gotten enough information from scans and blood tests to know that you must work on your immune system in order to heal, you may choose to join us in the Misner Plan, with your practitioner's input about your unique needs providing support and direction, and then simply watch the blood work and scans (MRI and color-Doppler ultrasound). If nothing changes (which is positive progress when it comes to cancer), or you begin to see interval improvement, your practitioner can monitor your progress so you will know healing is happening. There are even some oncologists who would be willing to monitor your condition during this phase of healing. All the better! Just don't be surprised if they say, "What are you doing again?" or "But you're not doing anything. How is this possible?"

The first thing we both did to start on our respective healing paths was to change our diet to greatly reduce sugar intake, including fruit sugars. Our first book, *Healing Begins in the Kitchen*, outlines our dietary changes and includes recipes with the approved foods list. The next thing we did was to begin using pancreatic enzymes. We both used P-A-L Digestive Enzymes, available online from Get Healthy Again and listed in the resource section. We took six enzymes on an empty stomach, four times per day during our active healing times. That is close to the maximum amount recommended. Third, we got organic Osage oranges (ordered from Amazon, believe it or not), cut them into quarters, froze them, and then grated 1 Tbsp. per person into our morning Sunshine Smoothie every day. You will find the recipe for this smoothie in *Healing Begins in the Kitchen*. Just making those changes brought a drop in Ivan's PSA from 12.8 to 7.4. Hedge apple powder is available now for those of you who do not have access to the fresh fruits, and there is a link for the online source in the resource section of this book. Those three things are easy to start right now, and they will help boost immune function right away. Again, please check with your healthcare practitioner regarding your specific needs.

Moving right into the next level of healing, we both focused on making sure to have time each day to do a quiet meditation, giving our bodies the chance to slip into a parasympathetic-dominant state. Adding a salt-water soak, breathing deeply while quietly focusing on gratitude, peace, and love while you are soaking will boost immune function even more.

Just doing these few things will help you avoid being overwhelmed and living in constant fear. Remember that when you allow your thoughts to race, imagining the worst and fearing the unknown, you are allowing your mind to suppress your immune system. Instead, focus on directing your mind to be your strong partner in healing: focus on how much you stand to benefit from the positive changes this health issue is bringing into your life, how grateful for each and every day you are, and then take time to receive all the love your friends, family, and business associates have for you.

BOOSTING THE
IMMUNE SYSTEM

Beth and Betty

Doing everything possible to boost my (Beth's) immune system was my primary focus during my time in the Healing Bubble. I did everything Dr. Christian Issels and Dr. Walter Kim recommended that I do and then some. When I had my second follow-up call with Dr. Issels after returning home, I shared with him that I was doing all he had recommended plus a bit more. He told me that I was almost doing too much.

"You can overtax your immune system, Elisabeth. It's possible to wear out the system by doing too much," he wisely cautioned. This counsel allowed me to back off and set a less intense pace of treatments I was doing at home, such as hyperthermia and colon hydrotherapy.

We (Beth and Betty) are going to share with you many things that can be done to improve immune function, but please be sure to work with your own healthcare provider before you apply these approaches into your own healthcare routine. You need to do what is indicated in your own case, not necessarily what I (Beth) needed to do. I will have a list at the end of each of the next two chapters for you to see what my own protocol included. You should work with your own integrative medical doctor, naturopathic doctor, or other doctor to build a protocol that will work best for you.

I used the approach of Dr. Issels, which is to focus on the entire body system, rather than singularly focusing on the tumor. Removing the tumor from the equation does not always keep you from developing other tumors. The tumor may have shed those circulating tumor cells (CTCs), which can begin to congregate in other organs, tissues, bones, etc. and form another tumor elsewhere. Dr. Issels' and others' approach is to create an environment in the body that maximizes the immune cells' ability to detect CTCs and eliminate them and also to make the body an inhospitable host for malignant growths.

If you want to be amazed, go to YouTube and search for videos showing microscopic footage of natural killer (NK) cells dismantling cancer cells. It's true that cancer cells can hide from immune cells, so it's important to boost the immune system and do the things that will weaken cancer cells, which will be our focus in the upcoming chapters.

This chapter covers physical techniques, supplements, and approaches for supporting the immune system. Again, we want to stress that before adopting these techniques, please find an integrative medical doctor, a naturopathic doctor, or a healthcare professional who practices functional medicine to guide you. There is a resource section at the end of this book that will give you the names and websites of some doctors you might wish to work with.

Physical Techniques to Boost the Immune System

Regulate Lower Bowel Function with Enemas and Colonics

The first priority in healing is the functionality and regularity of the lower bowel. It must be moving regularly and consistently to rid the body of toxins in order to prevent the reabsorption of those toxins from waste that sits in the bowels too long. Enemas and colonics are vitally important processes in all healing efforts. The difference between an enema and colonics is the amount of time and frequency of applications used in the therapies. Both methods use the principle ability of the lower colon to absorb and re-absorb liquids to quickly and efficiently provide the body with direct access to nutrients or hydration without having to involve the digestive processes. Colonics are beneficial for immune function and efficiency; modern science has identified that about 70-80% of the body's disease-fighting abilities originate in the digestive tract, specifically in the gut. Keeping the colon free of parasites, opportunistic microbes, and yeast is critical for a healthy immune system, and colon hydrotherapy helps with that.

Coffee enemas are usually held in the body for about fifteen minutes to facilitate the removal of toxins and prevent reabsorption and recycling of toxic bile, whereas colonics may use an irrigation of water repeatedly over a fifteen- to forty-five-minute span.

Coffee enemas are not some new, trendy, alternative medical modality. They were common practice in healing starting about 1500 BC. Until the 1970s, they were actually part of the standard of medical care listed in medical texts. The benefits include improved mental clarity, improved energy, relief of chronic pain, elimination of parasites, and improved digestion. A coffee enema can reduce discomfort experienced while detoxifying because the coffee eases the burden on the liver. The Herxheimer reaction (flu-like symptoms experienced when detoxifying) happens because the liver becomes overburdened as toxins move through the body, similar to how you may feel when consuming more alcohol than your liver can process.

Two specific components of coffee—palmitic acids called kahweol and cefestol palmitate—are absorbed into the portal vein system of the rectum, the lower portion of the colon, which leads directly into the liver. It is believed that these two palmitates enhance the glutathione S-transferase (GST) enzyme system. Glutathione is the body's primary detoxifying agent and is very beneficial in purifying the blood from known carcinogens. GST is the master antioxidant; it grabs on to toxins, binds them to reduced glutathione in the liver, and escorts them out of the body. The beneficial effect of palmitate in green coffee beans has been studied at the University of Minnesota by Lam, Sparnins, and Wattenberg, and it seems to stimulate glutathione S-transferase production *in vivo* up to 700%. More scientific study is needed in this area; however, there are many anecdotal cases of improvement, and even healing, after coffee enemas are included in a cancer-healing protocol.

Theophylline, another chemical compound in coffee, dilates blood vessels in the colon; this dilation enhances blood flow and improves muscle tone and therefore is believed to support tissue regeneration. The human body passes the entire contents of the blood supply through the liver every three minutes, so it is very important to keep the glutathione levels optimal. Anything we can do to reduce the burden on the liver is beneficial to the body's efficiency in healing itself.

Supplement with Beta Glucans

Beta glucans are key players in all efforts to strengthen and support immune function; they are immune system up-regulators. Beta glucans are polysaccharides (glucose polymers) from food-sourced fibers that equip the immune system to better recognize and attack foreign invaders and damaged cells, including cancer cells that need to be disabled and removed. As immune-boosting substances, beta glucans engage the immune system and complementary systems to inhibit tumor growth and protect against potential carcinogens. There have been many studies on the impact of beta glucans on immunity, many of which are available on the internet; they include results of studies that show beta glucans' ability to prevent oncogenesis and promote macrophage activation and NK cell cytotoxicity. Because the body does not produce beta glucans naturally, they must come from our food or in supplement form.

Beta glucan capsules can be taken orally with hot water (unless you use capsules from heat-extracted sources), but the powders may be more beneficial when made into suppositories by mixing them with liquefied cacao butter and coconut oil and poured into suppository molds that are then stored in the freezer for later use. Introduced into the body this way, the beneficial beta glucans can be delivered directly to your liver, bypassing the digestive system. We recommend 5 Defenders organic mushroom extracts blend made by Real Mushrooms, available online. When mixing the powders with the liquefied oils, wear a face mask to avoid inhaling the powders and irritating your lungs. Beth used these suppositories a couple of times per week at the rate of one per hour for six or seven hours per day in her intensive healing phase.

Natural food sources of beta glucans include oats, barley (a gluten grain), medicinal fungi (reishi, maitake, shiitake, cordyceps, lion's mane, and turkey tail, among others), yeasts, algae, and seaweed. We should point out that this immune-boosting substance is water soluble (effectively extracted with hot water), so it is best consumed in teas, broths, or coffee.

MGN-3, or Biobran, a type of beta glucan, is developed from hydrolyzed rice bran and has been clinically tested and found to boost immune function by 300%, according to a study presented (and subsequently published in a number of medical journals) to the American Association for Cancer Research by N. Ghoneum and G. Namatalla. MGN-3 contains arabinoxylane, another type of glucose polymer that is modified by an enzyme from the shiitake mushroom to create this product, sold as Lentin 1000 Plus from Japan, available online.

Stimulate the Thymus

Thymus tapping stimulates the thymus gland to release T-cells, immune cells that can help to keep immune function high. These powerful immune cells are produced by the bone marrow and mature in the thymus gland, which is why they are called T-cells. To do thymus tapping, first find your thymus gland, located just underneath the first few inches of your breastbone, which runs from the cleft between your collarbones down to the bottom of the central column of your ribcage. With your left or right hand, curve your fingers so your fingertips are held closely together and tap in the following rhythm: ONE, two, three; ONE, two, three, with a bit firmer thump on ONE than on two and three. This is a good technique to use in the throes of something you find distressing or upsetting or immediately after becoming startled. It is also good to do for ten minutes before falling to sleep each night. Your thymus gland normally releases new T-cells at about 10 pm, *if* you are asleep by that time.

Stimulate Lymphatic Flow

The lymphatic system is one of the keys to immune function. Dry skin brushing with a special, natural-bristled skin brush is especially beneficial to immune function. The lymphatic system is made up of glands and nodes. This system does not have its own flow mechanism, so it is important to stimulate the lymphatic pump in a variety of ways, such as exercise. The contraction of muscles can move lymph, the liquid that contains a type of immune cells called lymphocytes, around your body. Bouncing on the bottoms of your feet on a rebounder (or simply on the ground), and lymphatic massage, in addition to daily dry skin brushing are great ways to stimulate your lymph. This is one of the particular reasons that it is important that you be well hydrated so there is sufficient lymph that will flow when stimulated. Referring to dry skin brushing, some people use the mantra, "Brush toward the heart," but that is misleading. There are key areas in the body where the lymph drains into nodes, so you need to understand where they are and brush toward them. Please refer to our depiction of the body with arrows showing you how to brush your skin toward the nodes that drain into your veins around the body. [Figure 1.1 Illustration by Dorian Prin]

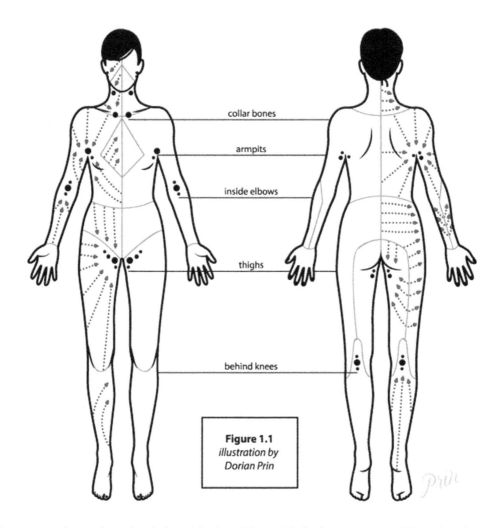

collar bones

armpits

inside elbows

thighs

behind knees

Figure 1.1
illustration by
Dorian Prin

Once you have brushed the skin briskly with light pressure (the glands are just under the surface of the skin and do not need to be vigorously stimulated to begin moving lymph), you can induce the nodes to begin draining into the veins by gently pressing or patting these areas of the body. The key spots are just below the collarbones, the armpits, inside the elbows, at the folds where your thighs crease when you bend forward, and behind the knees. It is also critical for women to stop wearing underwire bras, tight bras, and compression garments underneath all our clothes. These garments impede the flow of lymph in the body and simply create more congestion.

Take Salt-Water Baths

Salt-water baths draw much-needed minerals into the body to support immune function. Most people's bodies absorb up to two cups of whatever liquid the body is submerged into. If you do not have a whole-house filtration system on your water supply to remove chlorine from your bath water, run your bath a bit hotter than you want it to be when you get in, then let it stand for 15 minutes, the time it takes for chlorine to dissipate from your city water supply. It is important when taking salt-water baths, that the bath water not be extremely hot. Use Epsom salts (magnesium sulfate) or Dead Sea salts (also extraordinarily high in minerals), and soak for about 20 minutes. Avoid bath salts that are heavily perfumed, unless they contain pure essential oils only. Most scented Epsom salts contain "parfum," or fragrance, and not the actual essential oil; "fragrance" is a chemical you do not want to absorb through your skin. A daily salt-water bath can be a wonderful routine to establish that will really boost your immune function. Listen to music such as "Master Jack Lim's Inner Peace Relaxation" music, found on YouTube, during your soaking time. Master Lim embedded healing soundwave frequencies into this special music that is believed to impact your body at the cellular level and may support your own healing process. There are many other healing soundwave frequencies online you can play during your salt-water soaks. We suggest that you enter "Rife frequencies" as a YouTube search. You'll find a wide variety of healing tones that have a positive impact on the energetic vibrations your cells need for optimum vitality.

Supplements to Target Immune Function

There are particular supplements that target immune function. The most important are methyl B complex, folate, vitamin D_3, N-acetylcysteine (NAC), liposomal glutathione, and liposomal vitamin C. Below are descriptions of each of these supplements and their positive impacts on immune function.

Methyl B Complex

Methyl B complex is a methylated vitamin B complex that includes all of the B vitamins in a form that is easily metabolized by the liver. The term *methylated* has to do with the chemical composition of the supplement and the liver's ability to break down those compounds. About 30-50% of the population are non-methylators, which means they have the MTHFR gene mutation that leads to a lack of MTHFR enzyme production. We (both Betty and Beth) are in this category and lack the enzyme that would metabolize certain B vitamins such as folic acid and B_{12}. For non-methylators, taking a synthetic form of non-methylated B vitamin would cause additional stress on the liver and could be a contributing factor to our inability to heal. Most B complexes available in supplement form are derived synthetically, are often filled with excipients, fillers that are often indigestible, and put a strain on the body's natural processes. Vitamin Bs in general are important for metabolic functions, including the immune system and glutathione production. Vitamin Bs also help the body build up mineral reserves, assist in the stress response, and convert food to energy. As a side note, non-methylators benefit greatly from taking SAMe (S-adenosyl methionine) half an hour before eating. Please work with your own healthcare provider to determine if this would be beneficial for you and what your dosage should be.

Folate (Vitamin B9)

Folate, or vitamin B_9, deficiency can impair immune response, so when you focus on boosting immune function, you will want to be sure you have the ideal levels of folate in your system, and supplement if you need to. It is very important to work with someone skilled in biochemistry who is aware of your blood levels of folate. Excess folate has been implicated in some cancers, so balancing this micronutrient is important. Too much is not a good thing.

Vitamin D3

Vitamin D$_3$ is a steroid hormone that assists the body in immunomodulation. When introduced into the cell's DNA, D$_3$ initiates a cascade of molecular interactions that modulates sequence-specific genetic expression, specifically to affect mineral stores and boost the immune system. Vitamin D (1,25-dihydroxyvitamin D) is what the body manufactures from sunlight. The supplement form of vitamin D$_3$ is taken orally and is converted in the body to active form. It is recommended to take vitamin D$_3$/K$_2$ with menaquinone-7 (MK-7) and a meal including good quality fats. Often you may be able to find emulsified D$_3$/K$_2$, and this can be a good way to take this important micronutrient.

N-Acetylcysteine (NAC)

N-acetylcysteine (NAC) is an amino acid that is used in the body's manufacture of glutathione (discussed in detail next) in the cells. NAC is first converted to cysteine and then to glutathione. NAC is also used for any condition that involves mucous production and has been widely used as a supplement to support everything from neurological issues to immune function. Providing supplemental NAC may relieve some of the stress burden on the liver created by toxins.

Liposomal Glutathione

Every cell in your body manufactures glutathione. Glutathione is very important for detoxification as it protects the cell from free radicals that cause oxidative stress. Food sources or supplements of glutathione are not readily bioavailable, meaning that they are not metabolized well by the body. Glutathione molecules are too large to be absorbed through the digestive tract. This is the primary reason glutathione is given intravenously. It may also be nebulized for effective metabolism. Liposomal glutathione is glutathione that is coated with liposomes, the same type of material that human cell membranes are made of (phospholipids). The unique composition of phospholipids, or liposomes, makes it possible to keep glutathione in its reduced form, which is more bioavailable and stable. Liposomal glutathione can directly penetrate mucosal tissues in the mouth and throat, so it is protected from digestive juices and can more readily reach the liver, where it is then metabolized and released into the bloodstream to do its powerfully detoxifying work in support of immune function. A toxic body leads to a suppressed immune system. Non-methylators are especially susceptible to environmental carcinogens because they are glutathione deficient, as the MTHFR gene is one of three genes providing instruction for the cells to produce glutathione. In my (Beth's) case, this important gene is actually missing! There is a substantial segment of the population who are simply missing this gene. The Genova Diagnostics DetoxiGenomic test can determine if you are in this group. If so, you would most likely benefit from using liposomal glutathione a few times per day. Glutathione has a half-life of 14 minutes, so regular consumption of it throughout the day, rather than large doses once daily, is best for liver support.

Liposomal Vitamin C

Since vitamin C cannot be produced or stored in the body, it must be obtained from food sources. Vitamin C is a water-soluble vitamin needed for collagen production, immune function, bone health, and more. What the body does not use, it discards. The best way to get vitamin C into the body is intravenously (IVC) because it bypasses the digestive system and goes directly into the bloodstream when infused. As described above regarding liposomal glutathione, liposomal vitamin C may be taken orally to deliver this micronutrient directly in the bloodstream. Recent studies have shown the superior benefits to using liposomes to administer various nutrients such as vitamin C because of just how efficiently they are delivered to the blood stream using this carrier.

Support for the Immune System

Eat Green, Leafy, and Brightly-Colored Vegetables

Although many foods have been clinically studied and found to both boost immune function and to weaken cancer, our focus on boosting immune function is on green, leafy and brightly-colored vegetables. The Misner Plan (find the outline at www.MisnerPlan.com or in our book, *Healing Begins in the Kitchen*) gently moves your normal eating habits into a pattern that will support your immune system. Remember to include lots of leafy greens, and eat the rainbow!

Drink Liquids

Hydration is crucial for the proper function of the entire immune system. Water provides the needed conduit for the superhighways of your immune system to be wide open and flowing rather than congested and slow, like a highway during rush hour. The fastest way to bring your immune function to a screeching halt is to allow yourself to become dehydrated. While it is important not to drink too much coffee, tea, or other acidic beverages, they are not the primary cause of dehydration in the body. We nutritionists used to drill into our clients' heads, "Coffee is dehydrating." The science just does not support that. But anything more than two cups of coffee or black tea in a given day is going to create hyperacidity in your bloodstream, so your body will pull calcium from your bones in order to keep your blood alkalinity stable. Overconsumption of acidic beverages has been linked to osteoporosis. Acidosis is also a way to create a hospitable environment for cancer cell proliferation, since an acidic body is not going to be well oxygenated, either. Remember that water (H_2O) is bringing oxygen into your tissues!

To keep your body hydrated and your blood pH in the right range, set a goal each day to consume at least half your body weight in ounces of purified or (still) mineral water. We like to naturally alkalinize our drinking water with a squeeze of lemon. Lemons are high in minerals, and while they are citrus fruits—normally in the acidic category of foods, the minerals from lemons move the pH of purified water higher into the alkaline range. Still mineral water is naturally alkaline, while ½ tsp of Calm magnesium powder may be added to purified, filtered water to move the pH higher. In the case of a 135-pound woman, she needs at least 68 ounces of water each day in addition to coffee, black tea, juices, and any other beverages. Five 14-ounce glass water bottles would satisfy this daily requirement. You may count non-caffeinated, herbal teas toward your water intake if you do not add any honey to them. If brewed with dried, green stevia leaves, they may be counted toward your water intake.

If you don't like the way plain water tastes, you may add lemon or lime or even a drop or two of food-grade essential oil to infuse a nice flavor into your drinking water. Please don't drink water that has been stored in plastic water bottles. We will be discussing this in a later chapter. It is preferable to use glass drinking bottles for your daily water intake.

Take Low-Dose Naltrexone

Low-dose Naltrexone (LDN) is being used off label by some practitioners to induce serotonin production in the brain. Serotonin is an endorphin that serves as an immune function up-modulator. It is believed that LDN blocks this endorphin's effects on our bodies for a very short window of time (between 2 AM and 4 AM when taken at before bed), which causes the body to sense an endorphin deficit. The pituitary gland then signals for more serotonin to be produced. More serotonin throughout the day leads to higher immune function. There are no reported side effects from LDN. It is obtained by prescription from your doctor and must be compounded by a compounding pharmacist.

Promote Positive Feelings and Thoughts

Inducing "that healing feeling" through laughter, loving, philanthropy, and heart-warming stories (written and video) also stimulates neuropeptides and the production of endorphins that stimulate our immune function. This is the underlying principle behind Norman Cousins' "laughter therapy," through which he healed from his connective tissue disease and ankylosing spondylitis in the early 60s. These healing feelings stimulate the immune system. You will know the healing feeling when you get goosebumps, feel a lump in your throat, get a tear in your eye, or release a deep belly laugh. Dr. Mohammad encouraged me (Beth) to learn jokes and anticipate the joy I would get by making someone else laugh at my joke. That is a double blessing! Ask my husband and my kids. I started texting jokes to them and anticipating their positive reactions to the hilarity that ensued. Philanthropy also brings the healing feeling. It feels so good to serve someone else—to give from your heart in a way that is meaningful and life-changing to others.

Meditation and visualization are also two powerful techniques to boost immune function. When you engage in these two practices, you are triggering your parasympathetic nervous system. That brings your immune system fully online, and studies have shown that wounds heal faster, recovery from illness happens more quickly, and other body functions return to their optimal levels. The parasympathetic system helps us "rest and digest," two bodily functions we need working at the highest levels when healing and beyond. It is possible to have a very high-energy life and keep our immune function high if we make the time to have regular sessions of quiet meditation, contemplative prayer, and reflection—journaling, praying, or simply sitting still to regain our connection with the rhythms of nature and our natural environment. Most of us live with our sympathetic nervous systems dominant all day long, never moving into the important parasympathetic-dominant state. This is important for everyone, not only those who are healing.

Visualizations really kick up the body's ability to heal. We seem to be hard wired to induce healing by *imagining healing happening* in the body! When Ivan was diagnosed with prostate cancer, he printed out a large image of a dendritic cell and taped it to his computer monitor so that every time he glanced at that image, he could visualize this specialized cell moving through his body and signaling for T-cells and NK cells to come to the site of the prostate lesion and dismantle the damaged cells. I (Beth) did something similar by watching the "Big Red Tea Cup Bird Feeder" YouTube video and seeing in my mind's eye the lymphokine-activated killer (LAK) and Natural Killer (NK) cells "eating" the birdseed, which represented the cancer cells in my breast. Find the visualization that has the most meaning and works for you, and then do that visualization regularly.

Reducing and managing stress has already been thoroughly addressed in a previous chapter. It is a little-understood topic when it comes to boosting immune function by the general public. We all know we need to do manage stress better, but most of us really don't know where to start or what simple techniques to use. Stress is our natural mammalian response to change. In spite of all our technological advances, wisdom, spirituality, education, and scientific explorations and understandings, we are still biological animals with biological responses to change.

Change used to be threatening to our physical existence, and even though we do not intellectually realize it, this is how our bodies still respond to stressors. Our hindbrain, the reptilian brain we all still retain in this 21st century, responds to the stresses of our day in ways that suppress immune function. While it may not be possible in our lives to eliminate stress, as change is constantly happening, we can reduce change, and we can use the techniques available to us to manage the impact of change on our bodies, specifically keeping immune function high. We specifically endorse these techniques that reset your body's response to stress: the Heart Freedom Method, the Emotional Freedom Technique (EFT), meditation, exercise, qigong, and acupuncture (TCM). Knowing and practicing these techniques could mean the difference between a long, healthy life and a short, diseased life.

Spring Forest Qigong (SFQ) Five Elements practice is the final point of how to boost your immune system in this summary. Master Lin is so wise. He has traveled all over China, studying many different styles and forms of qigong under many qigong masters, and he has synthesized the most powerful aspects of many of them into his unique healing system. The SFQ Five Elements combines the physical movements and mental/emotional focus that maximize immune function. Each one of the five elements opens blocked energy channels and meridians, as wells as turns our attention to five higher values, or energetic signatures. These values switch on our immune systems as they trigger the neuropeptides that boost immune function: happiness, joy, peace, contentment, and gratitude. As you have already read, when I (Beth) was in my intense healing phase, I practiced this set three times per day. It was my lifeline, the core of my Healing Bubble. Now that I am once again healthy, I follow Master Lin's custom of starting each day with meditation followed by the SFQ Five Elements practice. On days that are challenging for me, I end the day with a shorter version of Master Lin's SFQ Five Elements.

Summary of Approaches for Boosting Immune Function

- ❖ Physical Techniques to Boost the Immune System
  - ➢ Regulate Lower Bowel Function
    - ▪ Coffee enemas
    - ▪ Colonics
  - ➢ Supplement with Beta glucans, especially via suppository
  - ➢ Tap your thymus
  - ➢ Stimulate lymphatic flow with dry skin brushing

> ➢ Take salt-water baths daily (Epsom salt or Dead Sea salt in warm, not hot, water)

- ❖ Supplements to Target Immune Function

  - ➢ Methyl B Complex
  - ➢ Folate
  - ➢ Vitamin D_3
  - ➢ N-Acetylcysteine (NAC)
  - ➢ Liposomal Glutathione
  - ➢ Liposomal Vitamin C

- ❖ Support for the Immune System

  - ➢ Eat green, leafy and brightly-colored vegetables
  - ➢ Drink liquids to stay hydrated (½ body weight in ounces of purified or still mineral water per day)
  - ➢ Take low-dose Naltrexone
  - ➢ Promote positive feelings and thoughts

    - ▪ Laughing—belly laughs and watching funny videos each day
    - ▪ Watching heart-warming movies, news clips, videos
    - ▪ Loving well
    - ▪ Philanthropy
    - ▪ Meditation
    - ▪ Visualizations
    - ▪ Reducing and managing stress
    - ▪ Qigong - Spring Forest Five Elements

WEAKENING CANCER CELLS

Beth and Betty

"But I want to know what the evidence is for alternative therapies and cancer," my (Beth's) dear friend insisted as we discussed her healing journey, which had followed the conventional path up to that point. She had been declared "NED" (No Evidence of Disease) twice in her journey and was facing more cancer, metastases that ended up invading her bones and lungs.

The good news is that the natural substances we will be discussing in this chapter *have been* clinically studied scientifically. They have not gotten the press the pharmaceutical "breakthroughs" have, and they often don't get the money invested in clinical trials that pharmaceuticals do because there is no money to be made in advising patients to eat broccoli, but they are often no less powerful and lack the serious side effects of most cancer-treatment medications. Dr. William Li, founder of the Angiogenesis Foundation, has invested a great amount of time, money, and research in phytonutrients that have been shown to have chemotherapeutic effects on cancer. You can read more about his work at www.eattobeat.org where you will find the research study reports on foods like watercress, green tea extract, stewed tomatoes, and watermelon. In addition, Dr. Siryaram Pandey, professor of biochemistry at the University of Windsor, has clinically studied the potential of dandelion root extract to exhibit powerful anti-cancer activity. These studies are so impactful that Ivan and I (Beth) have committed all the profits of our book sales and health coaching programs to

129

medical nutritional research. We want to support more of these types of research studies and clinical trials. The NIH (National Institute of Health) publishes many studies they have done which show the efficacy of natural therapies on cancer.

Some of the other therapies we will share in this chapter are being used with overwhelming success in other countries, but they are still unapproved by the United States' Food and Drug Administration for doctors to use to treat cancer. There are, however, no restrictions on US citizens to use these therapies on our own to weaken cancer cells. We cannot claim that they treat cancer nor that they can cure cancer. We are not suggesting that you use these therapies to treat cancer or cure cancer, but we are saying there have been robust scientific studies and clinical trials in many other countries that have shown these therapies' ability to weaken cancer cells enough that the body's natural defenses can do their job and return the body to homeostasis. We will share in the resource section of this book the names of doctors and clinics both in the United States and overseas where you may find clinically proven alternative treatment that is neither toxic nor carcinogenic.

In the meantime, we will share with you here what substances have been shown to have anti-cancer activity and are considered both anti-angiogenic and anti-tumoral.

Physical Techniques

Hyperthermia

The hallmark of the German cancer treatment protocols is hyperthermia, or induced fevers, typically by use of infrared sauna or focused infrared lights. Cancer cells are immature, mutated cells that cannot adjust to harsh conditions in the body, as mentioned earlier. Studies have shown, as reported by even the American Cancer Society, that fever-range whole-body hyperthermia may cause immune cells to become more active and raise the levels of cell-killing compounds in the blood. This treatment modality should not be used unless you are guided by a doctor who can set the upper limit of the temperature you should use for the length of time you need in order for the induced fever to weaken your cancer cells. That said, the German doctors, both alternative and conventional, as well as Ayurvedic doctors, have the longest history of using hyperthermia to treat cancer. It has been shown to be especially helpful when healing metastatic cancers. Hyperthermia is the underlying action in the FDA-approved prostate-cancer HIFU treatment (high focused ultrasound). Research also done by the Focused Ultrasound Foundation is available for review online, as is their listing of hospitals and clinics around the world using focused ultrasound (a form of heat ablation) both therapeutically and in clinical trials. Their website is www.fusfoundation.org. Fever baths, or induced fevers through the use of infrared saunas and infrared sauna blankets, is another way to utilize the healing power of hyperthermia to both stimulate immune function and weaken cancer cells.

Oxygenation

It has been clinically shown that cancer cells are linked to low levels of oxygenation in the body tissues. Dr. Otto Wahrberg won his first Nobel Peace Prize in 1931 for actually linking cancer to a lack of oxygen respiration in a cell. When clinicians who are doing research on cancer cells wish to halt the cell division *in vitro*, they routinely use oxygen to stop the cancer cells' multiplication. Cancer cells have difficulty dividing and multiplying in an oxygen-rich environment. This is the reason for seeking to saturate one's body tissues with oxygen in a hyperbaric chamber. Hyperbaric Oxygen Therapy (HBOT) is offered at quite a few cancer clinics now in the United States as part of integrative treatment plans; however, it does not have FDA approval for cancer treatment. It may be used as an adjuvant therapy. The advent of free-standing hyperbaric treatment clinics for enhanced sports performance, cosmetic improvement, and carbon monoxide exposure makes it much easier for the average person to have access at will to hyperbaric chamber treatments without the need for a doctor's referral. Again, we highly recommend that you seek your integrative medical doctor, naturopath, or other healthcare provider's instructions for how deep to "dive" and how long to stay in the chamber.

Deep-breathing exercises are critical to bringing healing to the body and weakening cancer cells. You have read above about the use of HBOT with cancer treatment, but did you know that you can have a huge impact on the level of tissue oxygen saturation by simply breathing deeply and intentionally for extended periods of time? We've all probably used or heard the phrase, "take a cleansing breath." One of the great strengths of relaxation practices such as qigong, t'ai chi, yoga, pranic healing, and meditation is the focus on deep breathing. This is true of exercise, too. Anything that gets you breathing deeply is going to have a positive metabolic impact. Shallow breathing or holding one's breath during times of stress or even simply answering email can restrict cellular access to oxygen. Watch your breathing patterns next time you are in your inbox. You may be surprised to realize how often you stop breathing briefly while dealing with email.

Cancer cells are simply stronger in an anaerobic environment. Be sure your body is experiencing aerobic conditions by doing deep-breathing exercises. Remember that each lung has multiple lobes, so imagine that you are breathing deeply enough to completely empty and refill each of the lung's lobes with every breath. Take breaths deeply enough to send fresh oxygen all the way down to the tips of the bottoms of each lung, passing through all the lobes. Then exhale so completely that you have facilitated a complete exchange of healing, oxygen-rich air. Know that every time you do this, you are sending more and more oxygen into your red blood cells where it will be moved into your body's tissues.

Dietary Changes

Cancer-Fighting Foods

Foods that have special cancer-weakening properties include raspberries for their ellagic acid (one cup of blended raspberries per day) and cruciferous vegetables (broccoli, cauliflower, cabbage, radishes, Brussels sprouts, and the like) for their sulforaphane and a whole host of other anti-tumor compounds. The two most powerful cruciferous foods are broccoli sprouts and watercress. We recommend eating them every day. An additional special food most people do not even have on their radar is the Osage orange. Known as the hedge apple or monkey fruit, the fruit of the Osage orange tree is high in the chemical tetrahydroxystilbene, which has been studied for its anti-angiogenic properties. Although not considered by most people to be edible, it is non-toxic to humans and has been used by many cancer patients to weaken cancer cells. You can find many more foods and the studies linked to their phytocompounds that are anti-angiogenic at www.eattobeat.org.

Fasting

Water-only fasting has been clinically studied by Dr. Valter Longo at the University of Southern California (USC). The conclusions of his studies have been fascinating and also definitive regarding the impact of water-only fasting on malignant tumors. As previously mentioned in my (Beth's) story, this modality is so exciting to the pharmaceutical companies that they are working to develop drugs that create the fasting-mimicking response in the body! Or, again, one could simply fast. This is a modality that requires the support and guidance of your healthcare practitioner. Since you are taking in nothing but purified water, your doctor should be the one to make sure you are in a healthy position to do this.

The science behind this modality is based on how plunging the body into an extreme, harsh condition in order to stimulate its repair and regeneration mechanisms works to cause tumors to shrink. The body does two things when facing starvation. It gets busy eradicating and removing any and all damaged cells. While in starvation, the body cannot afford to keep cells that are not functioning properly in the system because they will use valuable resources. This includes immune cells, so there may be a drop in immune function during the fast, but also cells with DNA damage (cancer cells) will be devoured by macrophages. Once the patient begins consuming food again, the entire body reboots the immune system, replicating fresh cells, including immune cells, from brand-spanking-new stem cells. Your entire body gets a regenerative boost after long-term fasting.

There are two ways to approach fasting: three-days with water only several times per year or more frequently when in the intense phase of healing with your doctor's supervision; or adhere to a fasting-mimicking diet, or FMD, where you consume no more than 500 to 1000 calories per day for a longer period of time, as directed by your healthcare professional. Dr. Longo recommends following the FMD for five days twice a month for longevity. You can read more about water-only fasting and the FMD in Dr. Longo's book, *The Longevity Diet*.

Ketogenic Diet

The ketogenic diet was recommended immediately to me (Beth) when I started my detox-and-rebuild treatments at the Issels Medical Center, as I have mentioned earlier. The Misner Plan lends itself well to the ketogenic diet; the only real adjustment I needed to make was to be sure that 80% of my calories came from healthy fats, and that I did not eat more than 50 net grams of carbs. As soon as the body shifts from burning glucose for energy into fat-burning mode, you are in ketosis. It was fortunate for me that I had some stored fat on my body. That made the transition a little bit easier. Going into ketosis helped me drop this stored fat pretty quickly while I was eating delicious foods like guacamole, water-packed olives, germinated and dehydrated nuts. I was very happy with the foods I needed to eat to remain in ketosis. One note about the ketogenic diet is that for cancer patients, consuming large amounts of animal proteins can be counterproductive. High consumption of animal protein is routinely linked to higher incidence of cancer development; growth hormones and the acidity of animal-source foods are both thought to be implicated as underlying factors for this link. While in ketosis, the main sources of animal proteins I ate were small fish, like sardines and herring, and organic eggs from pasture-raised, non-GMO-fed chickens. We urge you to work with your medical team to create the right diet needed for your condition.

Dietary Supplements

Proteolytic Enzymes

Proteolytic enzymes, also known as pancreatic or systemic enzymes, are vital when your focus is on weakening cancer cells. An enzyme is a substance that speeds up or initiates a reaction without damaging itself, so it can be used over and over again. Proteolytic enzymes help with the digestion of proteins (pancreatin), carbohydrates (amylase), and fats (lipase). Inflammation is the result of protein, or fibrin, floating in the bloodstream. C-reactive protein (CRP) is produced by the liver and is an indicator, or marker, for inflammatory diseases when analyzed by blood test. Cancer is considered an inflammatory disease. Taking proteolytic enzymes orally on an empty stomach helps the body to clean the blood stream and digestive tract of these rogue proteins and therefore reduces inflammation. The best time to take proteolytic enzymes is at night before bed, when the body is repairing itself during sleep. When taken with food, a broad-based enzyme supplement will help with the digestion of macronutrients consumed (proteins, carbohydrates, and fats) and will even help alleviate indigestion and reflux, as well as reduce inflammation in the body. When searching for a proteolytic or pancreatic enzyme supplement, it is important to find one that is broad based and includes as many types of enzymes as possible. Proteases are indicated by roman numerals: Protease I, Protease II, and so on. The Digest enzyme supplement used in the Misner Plan's Phase 1 is such a formula and is included in our detox kits, available at www.thehealthfixstore.com.

Enzyme therapy has been studied for decades relating to its impact on cancer cells. Dr. John Beard, an embryologist, first proposed in 1906 that the rapid maturation of the fetal pancreas and subsequent release of pancreatic enzymes, used to digest foods ingested long after birth, served a unique purpose early in fetal development regarding halting the rapid multiplication of the cells forming the placenta. He extrapolated that pancreatic enzymes could also be used to halt the rapid multiplication of malignant cells. Several case studies of his test subjects documented tumor regression and even complete remission from terminal cancer diagnoses after implementing his enzyme therapy. After Dr. Beard's death in 1923, his research was mostly forgotten. A Texas dentist, Dr. William Donald Kelley, used high-proteolytic-enzyme therapy with great success seventy years later with his patients who wanted to heal cancer naturally. Dr. Robert Good, the then president of the Sloane Kettering Institute, supported a case study of patients treated with the Kelley protocol. The results of the study were profound when narrowing the participants down to the ones who actually followed the protocol for the recommended amount of time. A number of them survived far beyond what could be expected, including one who lived over 20 years from her original diagnosis of pancreatic cancer to the liver. Both Ivan and I (Beth) have used pancreatic enzymes taken between meals on an empty stomach during our healing journeys. The specific product we used, P-A-L Enzymes, is listed in our resource section.

Another known benefit to using pancreatic enzymes to weaken cancer cells is that these enzymes help to dissolve, or digest, fibrin, as mentioned above. Cancer cells are shielded from the immune cells by a fibrin coating that is about 15 times thicker than the fibrin coating on normal cells. It is this extra-thick coating that allows the cancer cells to be invisible to immune cells—an invisibility cloak of sorts. As an added bonus, immune cells stimulated by proteolytic enzymes can produce even more chemical compounds that help them destroy cancer tumor cells.

A word of caution for those using blood thinners: the use of proteolytic enzymes can intensify the effects of anti-coagulants, so you should not add them to your own protocol or you will run the risk of bleeding. The same is true for hemophiliacs. While there are no known side effects in the general population from pancreatic enzymes, for these people, they are contraindicated and should NOT be used.

Magnesium

Magnesium is a natural substance that the body uses for over 300 metabolic functions, from muscle relaxation to energy transport. Work with your healthcare provider to determine the best type of magnesium for you and your dosage. It is critical to have enough magnesium in your body to assist in weakening cancer cells.

N-acetylcysteine

N-acetylcysteine (NAC) is a powerful antioxidant, as mentioned previously, that aids in the production of glutathione. Remember that glutathione is the body's master detoxifier and plays a crucial role in the immune function. We mention it again here for its ability to weaken cancer cells, as it is widely considered chemoprotective for its role in the protection of DNA.

Iodine

Iodine is most commonly known for goiter prevention and thyroid disease; however, when considered for its role in cancer protection and prevention, it is also anti-oxidant and anti-inflammatory. In addition, it plays a role in apoptosis (cell death) and cellular differentiation (the ability of cells to become specialized). Cancer cells are undifferentiated in nature, so achieving cellular differentiation within a tumor is a great success.

Vitamin D₃

Vitamin D has been extensively studied in recent years and has been found to have numerous mechanisms or activities that promote cell differentiation, reduce tumor angiogenesis (blood vessel formation), stimulate apoptosis, and decrease cancer cell growth. The Sloan Kettering Center has conducted quite a few studies that have shown Vitamin D to have treatment and preventative benefits to a variety of types of cancers, including breast cancer (Blackmore, Lesosky, Barnett, et al, and Robien, Cutler, Lazovich). For maximum absorption, we reiterate the need to use an emulsified (in a fatty carrier) form of D_3/K_2, or better yet, sunbathe as nude as you can be for ten minutes per day. It can also be helpful to provide the building blocks to vitamin D production, dietary cholesterol, prior to sunbathing. Simply eat an egg yolk, or a hard cheese before heading out to the sun. Do not shower for at least an hour after sunbathing to allow the vitamin D to be synthesized by your skin.

Vitamin C

Vitamin C has been studied specifically for its ability to create a hydrogen peroxide chemical reaction that may kill cancer cells. The National Cancer Institute (NCI) publishes results of studies at www.cancer.gov relating to intravenous vitamin C (IVC), concluding that treatment with high-dose vitamin C slowed the growth and spread of prostate, pancreatic, liver, colon, malignant mesothelioma, neuroblastoma, and other types of cancer cells.

In order to have the most therapeutic effect, high-dose IVC is best: from 75 to 100 grams. We found that we needed to ask specifically for non-GMO sources of IVC, such as from the cassava plant, rather than from genetically modified beets, which seems to be the source of most IVC.

Ginger

Dried, ground ginger stands alone in a class all by itself for its cancer-weakening capacity due to several phyto-chemotherapeutic components it contains, such as the most abundant chemicals, 6-gingerol and 6-shogaol. A study reported in *PLoS One*, a peer-reviewed, online journal published by the National Institutes of Health, recently showed that 6-shogaol is reported to be 10,000 times more effective than traditional chemotherapy in fighting breast cancer by inducing selective cell degradation. Normally healthy cells are not negatively impacted by 6-shogaol, but malignant cell degradation and eventual dissolution is induced by this naturally occurring chemical. Ginger has many chemoprotective and anti-inflammatory qualities and certainly should be a part of any cancer weakening protocol for its benefits, as well as its positive impacts on both digestive functions and detoxification of the liver.

Melatonin

Melatonin is the body's sleep and wake regulating hormone. The advent of the electric light bulb has forever changed our body's ability to efficiently produce this vital hormone. Wouldn't you know that melatonin has been clinically shown to weaken cancer cells? A study done in China at the Anhui Medical University by Zhang, Qi, Zhang, He, Zhou, Gui, and Yang on gastric cancer cells showed that melatonin "could inhibit cell proliferation, colony migration, and cellular efficiency . . . and it promoted apoptosis" (reported in *Biotechnic and Histochemistry Journal*). This hormone is excreted by the tiny pineal gland located approximately just above, behind, and between the eyes. The body takes naturally produced serotonin (the calming, awake, and alert hormone) and converts it to melatonin during the night. Artificial light interferes with this conversion and causes disruptions in sleep cycles. This is important to know, because the body does most of its repair and restoration during deep sleep. It is possible to supplement with melatonin, but it is best to retire to a darkened room (or use lights in the red/yellow color frequencies, candles, or firelight) about an hour before you plan to be sleeping.

Calcium D-Glucarate + Diindolylmethane (CDG DIM)

Calcium D-Glucarate + Diindolylmethane (CDG DIM) is a combination that supports hormonal balance in the body. Calcium D-Glucarate (CDG) alone is a substance produced naturally in the body and obtained through consumption of certain fruits and vegetables, such as cruciferous vegetables like broccoli, cauliflower, and cabbage. Through extensive studies, CDG has been shown to inhibit an enzyme found in certain bacteria that reside in the gut. This activity supports the body's ability to detoxify estrogens (important when healing estrogen-dominant cancers), foreign molecules, and fat-soluble toxins. It is not possible to consume enough fruits and vegetables to get enough CDG in a typical diet, due to the loss of nutrients in our food supply due to soil-mineral depletion, so supplementation will give you the highest concentration of CDG you can get.

Diindolylmethane is a natural estrogen modulator that deprives estrogen-dominant cancer cells of one of their primary energy sources. It is the primary metabolite, a chemical that supports the breakdown of indole-3carbonol, found in cruciferous vegetables like broccoli, Brussels sprouts, cabbage, kale, and cauliflower. When these vegetables are eaten and come in contact with stomach acid, DIM is formed in the body. DIM is not estrogenic, so it is widely researched for benefits with many types of cancer, such as breast, cervical and uterine. DIM supplementation helps to remove excessive estrogens from the body and balance out hormonal ratios.

Oils, Extracts, and Herbal Teas

Oils, both expeller-pressed and essential oils, can be your new best friends when you are focusing on regaining health after a cancer diagnosis: specifically, frankincense and German chamomile essential oils, along with CBD and bitter almond expeller-pressed oils. These oils have properties that are absorbed by cells with DNA damage and weaken them to the point where they can no longer multiply rapidly and expand into other tissues. The essential oils in particular contain terpenes that weaken circulating cells with DNA damage: malignant daughter cells and CTCs. These oils are best applied topically over the area where the tumors are located. We recommend Rocky Mountain Oils (RMO) for this purpose. I (Beth) made a blend of the essential oils (German Chamomile and Frankincense with bitter almond oil and a liposomal magnesium/MSM gel by Ancient Minerals, which helped the oils penetrate deeply into the tissue in my breast when I applied them directly over the tumor location. CBD oil is best used sublingually to weaken cancer cells. Legends Drops CBD oil is one of the most potent organically grown CBD oils we have found, and it's the one I used in my healing journey. We have listed RMO and Legends Drops in our resource section. Please work with your healthcare provider to determine the dosage appropriate for your condition.

Ingesting essential oils, including using them sublingually, should be monitored closely by a highly qualified and certified aroma therapist. Dr. Mohammad supervised Beth's oral use of German chamomile, oregano, and frankincense essential oils. We recommend consulting the National Association of Holistic Aromatherapy (www.naha.org) to find such a practitioner.

Certain plants have been shown to offer anti-cancer properties, and extracts are available that provide the healing properties to us. The most powerful tinctures (which are simply more concentrated extracts, usually extracted with alcohol) for weakening cancer cells are dandelion root, myrrh, bitter melon, and pau d'arco. Extracts and tinctures can be obtained from your healthcare provider. Typically, naturopathic doctors are best equipped to support your healing journey with these healing substances. If you are unable to find a naturopathic doctor or herbalist who can dispense these substances for you, you may use capsules, essential oils, or teas.

Green tea extract is another powerful cancer-weakening substance. Rich in EGCG, green tea extract may be taken in capsule form or in a tincture. You receive more of the phytochemicals when using green tea extract than simply drinking the tea.

Herbal teas have been used for centuries to weaken cancer cells. The most powerful anti-angiogenic teas are believed to be sour sop or guanabana (also called graviola) and Essiac tea. Essiac tea is a specific herbal blend created by Canadian nurse, Renée Caisse, who has been credited with helping many people heal cancer naturally. If you find this blend in a local herbal shop, be sure it contains French sorrel, as some blends are now missing that specific, healing herb. Graviola is also sold in capsule form as Ellagic Insurance with Graviola, available on Amazon. Dandelion root herbal tea can also be therapeutic to drink.

Laetrile

B$_{17}$, also called Laetrile, is seen as a selective anti-tumoral compound that targets only cancer cells, and it has been used for this purpose for many decades in many countries, including Mexico. Derived from apricot pits and bitter almonds, the substance amygdalin, a nitrioloside, resembles the B complex structure, so it was called B$_{17}$ by Dr. Krebb, who isolated this substance in 1952. For those who do not travel outside the United States for alternative therapy in order to receive Laetrile infusions or injections, bitter almonds and apricot pits are available at many natural health food stores. There are important, specific recommendations for how to best eat apricot pits to weaken cancer cells, since these seeds also contain small amounts of cyanide. We recommend that you work with your healthcare provider to establish the best way to eat them for your specific condition. With guidance from your healthcare provider, we feel the potential benefits far outweigh the dangers that allopathic doctors associate with Laetrile. When one considers the serious, systemic toxicity and carcinogenic nature of the conventional use of chemotherapeutic agents, the selective effect of Laetrile on cancer cells seems to be quite superior.

Using Relaxation for Weakening Cancer Cells

Visualization

Visualizations for weakening cancer cells were part of my (Beth's) practice. While there have been no large-scale studies on the ability of visualizations to weaken cancer cells, we have included it here because there are many studies that show a connection between the mind and the body, and many anecdotal incidents to support that connection. Master Lin's Cancer Healing meditation, available for download at www.SpringForestQigong.com, has one section where the meditators envision loved ones around them sending white light with great heat into the area of the body where there are cancer cells. As the meditators come to this part of the meditation, they visualize this white light getting hotter and hotter, heating up the cancer cells. I did a lot of visualizations of my beloved cells transforming and being released as energy. One visualization that I continue to do to this day is to breathe in pure, healing energy from the universe, from God. On the exhale, I visualize any energy my body does not need being released from my body like smoke from all parts of my body, especially from the breast where the tumor was. I continue this visualization until I see the smoke fading away and my exhalations are clear and pure. Another visualization called Ice, Water, Mist has a focus of seeing the malignant tumor encased in an ice cube. As the meditator watches the ice cube, it is seen in the mind's eye transforming into water, holding the mutated cells that need to transform within the water. The water and the cells are then visualized turning into mist and released from the body with each exhale.

Guo Lin Qigong

Qigong has been written about already, but we wanted to be sure it was included here in this chapter about weakening cancer cells. We encourage you to learn the Cancer Walk, or Guo Lin Qigong. Master Jack Lim has a beautiful video posted on YouTube that instructs us on all the elements of the walk, its history, its impact, and the process to prepare for the walk, how to do the walk, and the conclusion of the walk. This walk can be done for 45 minutes at a time, for several sessions each day, if you are actively healing cancer. Guo Lin Qigong is one of the first types of qigong that has been scientifically studied and has had its value medically proven, according to the Australian organization, Qi Gong Chinese Health. Most of the studies conducted at Beijing's Qi Gong and Cancer Research Unit of Guo Lin Qigong and other forms of qigong have linked the improved oxygenation of cells to the health improvements seen relating to cancer as it pertains to qigong healing potential.

Summary of Approaches for Weakening Cancer Cells

❖ Physical Techniques

144

- ➢ Hyperthermia
- ➢ Oxygenation
    - ▪ Hyperbaric therapy
    - ▪ Deep breathing exercises
- ❖ Dietary Changes
    - ➢ Cancer-Fighting Foods
        - ▪ Raspberries
        - ▪ Cruciferous vegetables
        - ▪ Broccoli sprouts
        - ▪ Watercress
        - ▪ Osage orange
    - ➢ Water-only Fasting
    - ➢ Ketogenic Diet
- ❖ Dietary Supplements
    - ➢ Proteolytic enzymes
    - ➢ Magnesium
    - ➢ N-acetylcysteine (NAC)
    - ➢ Iodine
    - ➢ Vitamin D
    - ➢ Vitamin C—high dose IVC
    - ➢ Dry, ground ginger
    - ➢ Melatonin
    - ➢ Calcium D-Glucarate + Diindolylmethane (CDG/DIM), specific to breast cancer
- ❖ Oils, Extracts, and Herbal Teas
    - ➢ Oils

- Frankincense essential oil (topically and sublingually)
- Chamomile essential oil (topically and sublingually)
- CBD oil
- Bitter almond oil

➢ Extracts/Tinctures

- Myrrh (tincture)
- Dandelion root extract (tincture)
- Bitter melon/pau d'arco extract (tincture)

➢ Herbal Teas

- Green tea extract
- Graviola (sour sop/guanabana) leaf tea
- Essiac tea
- Dandelion root tea

❖ B17/Laetrile
❖ Relaxing Support for Weakening Cancer Cells

➢ Visualizations
➢ Qigong

MANAGING
MENTAL HEALTH

Ivan

I have had the chance to write and speak from time to time about how to create balance in life, something Elisabeth has struggled with as long as I've known her. We both can see now how her tendency to pile more and more on her schedule negatively impacted her physical health by eroding her mental health. And this is true for many, many other people. While there are a wide variety of physical causes for a breakdown in immune function so complete that cancer is allowed to proliferate in one's body, there are also mental and emotional factors contributing to the rise of cancer.

Elisabeth's tendency to move toward burnout has contributed to her experience of being what she would call "out of control" of her life overall. And as an entrepreneur with many irons in the fire at the same time, I have certainly seen within my own life that finding time for family, business, and leisure time can be challenging. It's difficult to do it all.

Maybe you would like to know the secret to finding a way to balance. Am I right?

Forget about balance; it's an illusion.

Balance assumes that we spend an equal amount of time in all or most areas of our life. It is like the image of the scales where everything is completely and equally weighted and there is no movement. It assumes that we must spend a certain portion of each week devoted in some equal measure to every area that is important in our lives.

The problem is that almost no one can actually achieve that. We tend to live such hectic, busy lives that it is incredibly difficult to fit it all in. So, what do we do about this? For me, it's about creating *harmony*, not balance. This is more than semantics—it is a different way of looking at life. While life can't be fully in balance, it is possible to create a life that is in harmony with your vision of who you are and what you want to do. If that resonates with you—try the following simple techniques.

Wherever you are—be there. Here are three simple words that can begin to make a huge difference in creating harmony in your life: *be here now*. Wherever you are, be there. If you are at work, don't be thinking about the time you didn't spend with the family the night before or what you should be doing with your significant other right now. When you are at home, don't be thinking about the work you have to do at the office. Wherever you are, be there, fully and completely. When both Beth and I were healing actively, it was so important to really live this mantra until it became a habit. Now that we have recovered our physical health, this aspect of sound mental health remains a constant for us.

Be creative about how you manage your time. If you have a big project at work that has to get done and you also want to spend quality time with the family one evening—get creative. When I was writing my first book, I used to spend the evening with the family, and once everyone went to bed, I sat down to write. I finished the book without taking any time away from the family. Be creative and inventive in finding ways that you can accomplish what you need to do yet still allow you to spend time doing the other things in your life that bring you harmony. For Beth, this means metaphorically "singing." When I came in the kitchen one day during her healing journey, I was so touched to literally hear her singing. It had been years since I had heard her voice lifted in song. I knew she was finding harmony in her life again.

Integrate the various elements of your life. For many years, I spent a couple of weeks or more working remotely from our lake house. Over time, I began to bring our company's global support and management teams up to the lake for short offsite retreats. It was a great way to combine my work life and a leisure environment. Afterwards, I took time off completely and spent it with the family. By integrating my two worlds, I created a sense of harmony. Look for ways to integrate these different elements of your life whenever possible.

Practice letting go and holding on. Contrary to popular belief, I do not think it is possible to have it all. Unfortunately, life involves making choices. Practice understanding what things to say no to and then letting go of them. At the same time, think about the things that are truly important in your life, and then hold on to them with all of your might. For Beth, this meant that during her healing journey she needed to let go of a lot of things in order to invest the time needed to do the home therapies and create enough space in her day-to-day so that she had the time to practice her t'ai chi forms, learn new qigong routines, write poetry, and do the other things that helped her re-orient herself toward healing. Once given the all clear, she has had to really watch her calendar so that she does not hold onto the things that drain her energy or bring her overmuch stress. Some stress is unavoidable, but sustained stress without any times of simply being quiet and creative does not help her stay healthy.

Be intentional about who you let in your room. Imagine that you live your entire life in one room, and that room has only one door—an Enter Only door. Anyone who gets in is there for life. If that were true, would you be more selective about who you let into your room? Everyone I ask that question answers with a resounding, "Yes!" Well, luckily this is only a metaphor; however, when we do let people into our lives that are caustic or difficult, it is very difficult to get them out. If you want harmony in your life, be more selective about who you let in your room. What I have watched my wife do is to become really sensitive about which new acquaintances seem to come with additional drama. Prior to her healing journey, she could not resonate with this metaphor at all. She actually said to me, "My room does not even have walls, much less a door!" And she was right. But it was that sense of openness that created a situation for her that found her dealing with a fair number of people who were high strung, whose lives were filled with drama that unfortunately spilled over into her heart, creating chaos for her, too. If you were to ask her about her room today, she would say that she now has walls, a door, and a good doorman. She has learned the wisdom of this concept of "who's in your room?"

Create margins. Life for most of us is crazy-busy. Create a life that has margins. Build in free time, family time, and personal time into the margins of your day-to-day existence. You'll be happier for it, I promise, and that will translate into better health. While you may think this is the same concept as creating harmony, it's a bit different. I am proud of how my wife has applied this concept. The changes she has made in this aspect of her daily life is inspiring.

Beth used to cram her every waking hour into a frenzied schedule. That schedule might have included time for charity work, time for her professional role, time for the family, and time for her artwork—all things she loved doing, but it did not allow much time for the margins.

The margins are where you simply slip into idle from going full-speed ahead. It's the space between appointments, the time where you breathe, or allow enough time to get from point A to point B that you have the space to stop by the roadside to watch two hawks playing in the updraft of a huge dust devil. Give yourself the gift of these margins, and stand back and marvel at what can happen in this space that will feed your soul, which in turn up-modulates your immune function.

Work in your flame not your wax. When you are doing things you resent doing or that you do out of compulsion, you are in your wax. You are doing things that are sapping your energy. When you are doing the things that you love to do, you are in your flame. You are energized and excited. If you want harmony, strive to do more that is in your flame and less than what is in your wax. Of course, there are things you must do in order to do what you want to do. Beth and I have both found plenty of those things hanging around in life. But when working in your wax dominates your life, you have discovered a sure-fire way to suppress immune function. Just thinking about it can cause adrenaline, a stress hormone, to flow.

I watched Beth let the things that were her wax dominate her days. And when I would point them out, her response came from the place of having her energy sapped—she was not receptive to my observations at all. She acknowledged my concerns but continued to go flat out. It was only after her healing journey ended that she could look back and see the damage to her health that working primarily in her wax had done. We share so honestly with you here to encourage you to identify for yourself where you may also be in your wax more than your flame. How can you shift this for yourself? It's so important to do. Please don't wait for a similar situation, a crisis like Beth's, to prompt you to evaluate your own life.

The truth is that when you are 70 years old, you are not going to wish you had spent more time at the office, in traffic, or struggling to meet deadlines. Not seeking harmony in your life is a great prescription for ending up in that same heart-to-heart conversation with your doctor that Beth and I have both had. Focus on creating harmony in your life. Be creative. Find ideas that work for you and the life you live. Make the time and be innovative. Harmony is created where harmony is sought.

ADAPTOGENS

Betty

We are including this information in our book because understanding how important these special herbs are for improving immune function and helping your body heal easily is critical. Beth used some of these herbs in her healing journey with my direction and the guidance of her medical team, and we want you to know about them.

Before I began my holistic practice over 15 years ago, I was searching for answers for my own health and for my son's. Under the guidance and support of a skilled naturopath, I replaced the twelve medications that he and I both were taking for various diagnoses with specific vitamins, minerals, and single herbs that are commonly used to control symptoms. Although this was a more natural approach, it was not optimal because I was still trying to control symptoms instead of correcting and restoring true health at the root level. The herbs and nutraceuticals were working overtime to restore adrenal strength and rejuvenate our immune systems. Although we experienced dramatic and lasting improvements in our health, the most profound improvements were seen when I was introduced to a specific class of herbs called adaptogens.

Just as the name implies, these special herbs confer adaptive properties to our health. They efficiently support many systems simultaneously in the body that other, more commonly used herbs could not address alone. The original criteria for this class of herbs was first defined by Dr. Nikolai Lazarev in 1947. In simple terms, adaptogens are herbs that meet your body where it is and provide vital nutrients to help the body master the stress response.

Although they have been used for centuries in TCM and Ayurveda, the recent successful use of adaptogenic herbs in the United States, combined with the broad scope of how they can support many systems within the body, is bringing the attention of allopathic doctors to their healing characteristics and benefits. It is much easier now to find clinical research on herbs for medicinal purposes, because they are being tested in hopes of synthesizing new medicines to cure and treat chronic degenerative diseases. There is a resurgence of interest across the globe in plant-based therapies, and the World Health Organization reports that 75% of the world's population is dependent upon some form of botanical medicine for basic healthcare needs. In fact, 25% of all pharmaceuticals in the US are still derived from plants that were once used in traditional medicine.

Adaptogens are considered the *elite* class of botanicals within the herbal community because they contain so many properties for the protection of the neurological and immune systems. Their other benefits include command of the stress response, anti-aging, prevention of chronic and degenerative disease, restoration of cognitive function, restoration of depleted and over-burdened body systems, and support of various metabolic functions.

Adaptogens help restore balance and homeostasis to the body and all systems—structural, digestive, endocrine, lymphatic, hepatic, renal, neurological, respiratory, pulmonary, and immune. These benefits also include restoration of energy, stamina, endurance, and efficiency of metabolic processes, without the letdown or crash of stimulants, which makes these herbs extremely powerful and useful for many people with varying weaknesses and conditions.

In 1968, Israel I. Brekham, Ph.D. and Dr. I. V. Dardymov formally gave adaptogenic herbs a functional definition that provides us with a better understanding of how these elite herbs are different. To paraphrase their technical definition, here are the main points:

- An adaptogen is nontoxic,

- An adaptogen creates a nonspecific response in the body in resistance to multiple stressors, and

- An adaptogen does not negatively affect the person or systems of the body.

The best and most concise way to describe the benefits of adaptogens is to use the terms *balancing* and *restorative.* These characteristics point us to an understanding of how they can act as homeostatic metabolic regulators, which is important as we further discuss the six specific herbs that qualify as primary adaptogens. It is worth noting that TCM and Ayurveda have a broader range of 18-20 herbs that classify as adaptogens.

The six primary adaptogens are listed below with brief explanations of their functionality in the whole body. There are also secondary adaptogens that compliment and support the actions of the primary adaptogens when combined and prepared properly. Adaptogens work most effectively when combined with other herbs, specifically secondary adaptogens and nervines (plants used to calm nerves). A few great partners are skullcap, all the beneficial mushrooms, cordyceps, lemon balm, St. Johns' wort, magnolia bark, and so many others. For the sake of space, we will only address the primary and a few of the secondary adaptogens that are especially beneficial in building immunity and supporting the endocrine-immune system in weakened states such as cancer and degenerative disease. The Misners used quite a few of these plants in their respective healing journeys.

The book, *Adaptogens in Medical Herbalism* by Donald R. Yance, CN, MH, RH (AHG), and the website http://adaptogensbook.com/ contain a *Materia Medica* (latin for medical material) that I go to often as my primary resource about adaptogens.

Primary Adaptogens

Ashwagandha

Ashwagandha is the most sought-after adaptogen when dealing with the endocrine system (the glands that produce all the various hormones in the body). It is excellent for building and tonifying the glands, especially in those of us who are exhausted or find ourselves in a weakened state. It boosts immune function and nourishes the cells. Ashwagandha, like all adaptogens, is best taken regularly for the long term. Ashwagandha is a root and is best prepared as a tea by combining one teaspoon of dried root powder in two cups of liquid and simmering together, covered on low heat, for 15 minutes. This results in a strong extract that you can sip on as Beth did regularly. Ashwagandha does best when its properties are extracted in fatty milk like coconut milk. It makes for a particularly effective herbal tonic when you combine this particular adaptogen with a nervine for a balancing effect. Your herbalist or naturopath should be able to direct you to the nervines best combined with ashwagandha, such as St. John's wort.

Astragalus

Astragalus membranaceus (*leguminosae*) has been reported to possess anti-tumor and immunomodulatory properties. It is also antiseptic, diuretic, and antispasmodic and relieves discomfort from gas. Its fern-like leaves are traditionally used to treat infections of the mucous membranes in the body. It is said to rejuvenate digestive organs and help with blood glucose levels. Commonly used in therapies for edema and diabetes, it has been shown to stimulate the activity of the white blood cells. This is why Dr. Issels recommended it to Beth. Astragalus is typically combined with other primary and secondary adaptogens. When you think of astragalus, it is helpful to imagine the fortification it brings to the body's defense mechanisms.

Siberian Ginseng

Siberian ginseng (*eleuthero senticosus*) is a bitter herb, adaptogenic, immune stimulating, and great for the circulatory system. It is used to enhance endurance, regulate blood sugar, and stimulate immune function due to its saponins, called eleutherosides. They work to increase the activity of NK cells, as well as other hormones and beneficial chemicals in the immune system. Eleutherosides also increase the efficiency with which oxygen is delivered to the cells, which makes them an excellent choice for use with aerobic exercise. With the use of eleutherosides, NK cells are mobilized and activated up to twenty-four hours after exercise ends, instead of the normal two hours. With any of the ginsengs, start with a low dose and work your way up gradually. Siberian ginseng is best at helping to raise cortisol levels when taken early in the morning.

Panax Ginseng

Panax ginseng is considered a "panacea" in TCM, as it is not used specifically to treat illness but rather to improve general well-being. It is tonifying and generally healing and is thought to move the body into a more favorable state. It contains a complex mix of triterpenoid saponins, glucosides that stimulate the midbrain, heart, and vessels, as well as the central nervous system. It is specifically used with the elderly and for those with weakened constitutions in order to restore vitality and strength. Panax ginseng is very effective as an aid to digest and metabolize free fatty acids for fuel, instead of glucose. It also helps to restore and reinforce circadian rhythms upon waking. You can see why it is helpful during times of healing and beyond.

Rhodiola

Rhodiola rosea, or golden root, has been studied by researchers Thomas B. Walker and Robert A. Robergs in Eastern Europe for its effects on fatigue, both physical and mental. Patients in these studies reported having more focus and energy. It was observed that both human and animal experimental models showed better endurance when supplementing with rhodiola. It is best to take rhodiola before eating. One thing to consider when supplementing with rhodiola is that it may cause a stimulating effect for some people, so we recommend you take it first in the morning and/or before lunch until you know how it will interact with your particular physiology. Beth used a tincture of Rhodiola rosea three times per day.

Schisandra

Schisandra chinensis is a plant that contains specific lignans in its berries. These berries are of particular interest to medical scientists for their medicinal value. It is a bitter adaptogen, expectorant, central nervous system depressant, and liver detoxifier. It supports the immune, nervous, respiratory, and digestive systems. Traditionally, it was used to suppress coughs and support respiratory functions, but since it shows hepatoprotective effects (protects the hepatic system components—parts of digestive system, liver, and portal vein) by increasing the enzymatic metabolism of toxins in the liver and increasing the production of digestive enzymes, it has been shown to improve the body's metabolic ability to eliminate toxins. It is best used in combination with stress-relieving herbs and adaptogens.

In my practice, I use Solle Naturals brand adaptogenic herbal formulas because they are easily accessible and quite economic. The adaptogens in these products are combined specifically to reduce inflammation and to target the endocrine system and are in premixed, powdered drink form without excipients or fillers. I have not found any brand other than Solle Naturals that utilizes the philosophy of the body-mind connection in their formulas as extensively and as purposefully to feed the neuroendocrine system. My clients have had much success with these formulas in rebuilding and restoring energy, stamina, and endurance to their endocrine-immune systems. I would encourage you to explore these formulas at www.sollenaturals.com and pay close attention to the herbal adaptogenic combination in Solle Vital, which contains all six of the primary adaptogens in high potency combinations. These products are Misner-Plan approved, and are used by both Ivan and Beth. They travel with Thrive, as well as Solle Vital.

Adaptogens and Supporting the Immune System

Adaptogens are the foundation of herbal immune-system revitalization efforts. They can either activate or deactivate messengers involved in the body's natural stress responses. They are safe for long-term use and can significantly improve cellular metabolism. They fortify the immune system by enabling the body to properly dispose of oxidative waste and reduce free-radical damage in the cells. Adaptogens also improve digestion of fats, sugars, and proteins, due to the fact that they also contain carotenoids, flavonoids, and phytosterols—phytonutrients that improve cellular energy production and promote anti-inflammatory action in all systems of the body. They actually aid in all areas of immune function: modulation, regeneration, rejuvenation, restoration, and recovery.

Adaptogens are powerful and necessary components of immune system support, especially when healing cancer naturally, like the Misners have both done. One of the keys to working with adaptogens is normalizing any abnormalities in the hypothalamus, pituitary, adrenal, thyroid (HPAT) axis by balancing hormones and engaging their protective properties to all systems. What I love about adaptogens is the simple way they rebuild body chemistry at the cellular level. I like to use the metaphor of a kitchen pantry when describing how they restore mineral and phytonutrient balance to the body. Think of it as having a full, bountiful pantry full of colorful, flavorful foods that are bioavailable to you at any time. In that pantry is a plethora of beneficial and powerful phytochemicals that are ready to strengthen and protect you on a moment's notice.

The role of adaptogens in cancer prevention and treatment is exciting due to recent discoveries and studies that are providing a wealth of information pertaining to anti-tumor properties and reversal of premalignant conditions. Adaptogens inhibit invasion, metastasis, and angiogenesis, and they increase the body's ability to adapt entire systems to cope with the demands of physical stress. Stimulating immunomodulation, these power-house herbs help the body activate and adapt macrophages, NK cells, antigen-dependent T lymphocytes, and interferon, a protein released by cells in an inhibitory response to viruses.

Basically, cellular communication is enhanced greatly when adaptogens are used in conjunction with other phytonutrients to optimize gene behavior. Using them in conjunction with single herbs, and the sound nutritional basis of the Misner Plan as presented in *Healing Begins in the Kitchen,* doubles and triples the benefits to the body during the cancer-healing process. These benefits include strengthening the overall health of the patient, increasing the efficiency of digestion and all bodily functions, increasing tolerance to radiation and chemotherapy (when that may have been the chosen treatment), providing general antioxidant protection from oxidative stress, slowing the development of other cancers, preventing metastasis, nausea, and fatigue, and finally, protecting vital organs in the body.

Adaptogens and the BodyMind

The concept of the mind and the body as truly one, inseparable unit is not a new idea. In fact, this approach dates back to the beginning of time until the 1700s when scientific discovery began, and emerging scientists were trying to make a name for themselves. Body systems were isolated and treated as independent factors in disease and sickness. In the 1800s when the microscope was invented, the *germ theory* was born. The world had an explanation for disease and disharmony that trumped the responsibilities of self-care and keeping the terrain (the body) inhabitable for disease. As the germ theory took hold, the world began to understand and assign a separatist view to the reality that food rotted for an explainable reason and to view disease as strictly due to pathogenic bacteria and viruses. We became complacent and comfortable with eating poorly and then taking medicines, all to the detriment of our body's terrain. Western medicine discarded the practices of TCM, Ayurveda, and traditional naturopathy and accepted the hypothesis of splitting the human being into two distinct and unrelated units: the mind and the body.

In the last twenty years, modern medicine has drifted far away from the thought of disease being significantly influenced by emotion, thought, belief, and spirituality. What was called the golden age of herbal medicine in the 50s and 60s is starting to emerge as a dominant factor in integrative and functional medicine, especially regarding chronic and degenerative diseases such as cancer. We are starting to see solid documentation of the body-mind connection in scientific evidence through research in the areas of neuroscience and epigenetics.

The truth is that science does support the body-mind connection by definition and always has. The neuroendocrine system is at the center of this complex, yet intricate, system of hormones and neurochemicals. By supporting the physical components of the neuroendocrine system with adaptogens, we are also able to target and support specific weaknesses in mindset, thought, perception, general outlook towards life, depression, chemical imbalances, and more. In my practice, I have seen permanent and lasting changes for the individuals who have started out in the throes of deep depression, only to suddenly emerge from the clouded perceptions of distrust, self-hatred, and feelings of not being enough after beginning a protocol of adaptogenic herbs. I do not hesitate to say that I have experienced miracles in my clients when it comes to the body-mind connection, and I am so grateful for these amazing herbal tools.

The immune system gives us the best example of the prevalence of this connection between body and mind as scientists have found specific receptors on the surface of immune cells that act like key-holes to certain chemical neurotransmitters released by the nervous system and the brain. These hormones are released and mediated by the autonomic nervous system (ANS) and are the key messengers in the cellular communication of the BodyMind.

We have talked about the release of certain neurotransmitters and hormones throughout this book. We want you to see the reality of the entire human body as a complex super highway of communication and influence with multiple, intricate pathways and connections to all systems, organs, and body functions. There is no separation of the body and the mind. To attempt to separate these two aspects of our existence would result in catastrophic effects on the entire collective system. The best approach, the *wholistic* (holistic + whole body) approach, is to properly nourish both the mind and the body simultaneously with synergistic and complementary herbal nutrition such as adaptogenic herbs. This is the only way to ensure optimal wellness, which is our goal, after all.

ADAPTOGENS AND THE ENDOCRINE SYSTEM

The endocrine system is made up of the hypothalamus, pineal, pituitary, adrenal and thymus glands, lymph nodes, spleen, bone marrow, and various white blood cells. It is the first line of defense in times of physiological stress. The endocrine system and the central nervous system work in concert to engage the adaptive response of the body by utilizing these glands to continually release hormones into the blood stream. The body responds quickly—think how fast the fight or flight response kicks in—but just because the threat ends or is removed, the body still must respond to the negative feedback loops created by the cascade of hormones and neurochemicals in order to restore itself to balance. The endocrine system takes the hardest hit from chronic stress as the long-term effects wreak havoc on the balance in this system. Endocrine exhaustion impairs the body's ability to adapt and recover efficiently. So many people experience daily fatigue and an overall lack of energy. It is the number one complaint among my clients, and it is also usually the number one focus in their minds when they consult with me. There is a reason so many energy drinks are being sold: people are starving for energy because their cells are not able to function properly to produce ATP, the energy currency of life, and their adaptive responses are depleted literally on the cellular level.

When the endocrine system is taxed beyond its means, the cells' energy-transport mechanisms suffer, mineral stores are depleted, and the stage is set for disease and tumor growth. This is where our perceptions, experiences, and mindset can physically and biochemically influence how our bodies respond to stress. Certain conditions must be present for the entire body system to function at peak efficiency, and unfortunately, it is quite easily disrupted by not only mental and emotional stress but also by environmental stress from toxic substances.

These chemical environmental stressors called endocrine disruptors are critical to know about and avoid as much as humanly possible. The most common and prevalent chemicals that disrupt the endocrine system are called the "dirty dozen." These twelve hormone-altering chemicals are: BPA, dioxin, atrazine, phthalates, perchlorate, fire retardants, lead, arsenic, mercury, perflourinated chemicals, organophosphate pesticides, and glycol ethers. Contamination with these toxins is experienced through inhalation, skin absorption, and ingestion, so protection and self-care are imperative to avoiding further environmental stress.

In the Misner Plan, we recommend these ingredients be eliminated from our routines, but the FDA considers them safe at the present time. The FDA claims there is no reason to be concerned, but we have learned to err on the side of being overly conservative in order to recapture and maintain our health. Some of the dirty dozen (such as BPA and phthalates) are slowly being removed from the food stream and certain products, but other products still contain them, and most of us are not even aware of it. For example, the thermal paper used for credit card receipts is coated with BPA, which is readily transferred to our fingertips and then can easily be absorbed through the skin or transferred to the mouth and ingested.

Following is a section on specific endocrine disrupters and what the studied physical effects have been in on the human body. We think you will be greatly enlightened by this section if you have not already researched these pesky substances. And we also suspect you might become overwhelmed or disheartened when you read how prevalent these substances is in our environment, in the products we use on a daily basis, and even the products we use when caring for our babies. We don't want you to lose heart. You can protect your body from the negative effects of these toxic substances, healing the body and staying completely healed. Knowledge is power, and we want to empower you to make substitutions where you can to reduce the amount of environmental stressors in your daily lives.

Chief Offenders of the Endocrine System and other Suspected Toxins

Chemicals are regulated by the Toxic Substances Control Act unless they are used as pharmaceuticals. The FDA regulates chemicals used in medicines and drugs. There are no testing requirements on chemicals used in personal care products as a rule, and no pre-market safety tests are required. As the cosmetics and personal-care industries grow and the health consciousness of the public expands, marketing tactics become more creative. Many known carcinogens and highly suspicious chemicals are still a part of the formulations of nail polish, shampoo, hairspray, lotions, soaps, and deodorants, among other products, but are camouflaged by new and different names.

The ways these chemicals enter our bloodstreams are varied but include absorption through the skin, inhalation, and ingestion. If you put products containing these chemicals on your skin (e.g. lotions, shampoos, and makeup), inhale them into your lungs (e.g. from hairspray, perfumes, and scented laundry detergents), or use them in your mouth (e.g. toothpaste and mouthwashes), the chemicals end up in your bloodstream where they may have a devastating impact on your liver. The liver is your strong ally in boosting immune function as it performs its powerful detoxification duties. Some chemicals are bio-accumulative, and still others are directly toxic to living things, although our governmental agency has deemed them Generally Regarded as Safe (GRAS) for human use. It is almost unheard of for a chemical used in personal care products to be restricted once it has already been deemed as GRAS.

But these same chemicals are known to be endocrine disrupters, causing a breakdown in a very important system your body relies upon for health: the hormonal system. Hormonal imbalances are responsible for many illnesses and certainly for a number of cancers, specifically breast and prostate cancer, as well as thyroid cancer, lymphoma, and others.

It is so important to your health, both in healing and preventing disease, to keep these hormone-disrupting, toxic chemicals out of your body as best you can. Somewhere along the way, we accepted that these chemical-laden blends were somehow necessary for personal care and hygiene. It's not true. Nature provides many single-ingredient substances that work just as well and may be used as inexpensive replacements for the toxic combinations found in your bathroom cabinet, makeup palettes, and laundry rooms.

We have listed here a few of the common offenders and their aliases that are used in cosmetics and personal care products to aid you in your efforts to detoxify your body and your home. In the next section, we are going to share recipes for replacements for many commonly used products that contain these chemicals. As much as you can, we recommend that you eliminate all products containing these chemical ingredients as part of the Misner Plan.

Formaldehyde, also known as:

quaternium-15

DMDM hydantoin

imidazolidinyl urea

diazolidinyl urea

sodium hydroxymethylglycinate

2-bromo-2-nitropropane-1,3 diol

glyoxal and oxaldehyde

formalin

formic aldehyde

methanediol

methyl aldehyde

methylene glycol

methylene oxide

polyoxylmethyl urea

sodium hydroxymethylglycinate

bromopol

glyoxal

These substances are already banned in Japan and Sweden and highly restricted in the EU and Canada. Formaldehyde and formaldehyde-releasing preservatives are found in nail polish, liquid baby soaps, shampoo, nail glue, synthetic or acrylic nail powders, body wash, color cosmetics, hair smoothing products, eyelash glue, and hair gel. These products are highlighted by the Campaign for Safe Cosmetics, reported by them to contain formaldehyde and formaldehyde-releasing preservatives.

Sodium lauryl sulfate, aka sodium dodecylsulfate, sodium lauryl sulfate ether, lauryl sulfate sodium salt, hydrogen sulfate, sodium salt, carsonol SLS, and dehdyrag sulfate GL emulsion. (Sodium laureth sulfate is made from sodium lauryl sulfate and is a distinctly different chemical but is also avoided in the Misner Plan). Sodium lauryl sulfate is found in a wide array of household cleaning products. It is commonly used as a detergent, but it has also been widely used in toothpaste, hair color, pet care products, marshmallow products, fresh fruit coatings, ready-made egg white emulsions, and as food additives and coatings.

Mineral Oil, aka liquid petrolatum, heavy mineral oil, white oil, liquid paraffin, and sunpar paraffins. This byproduct of the production process that turns oil into gasoline is used as a lubricant or laxative. Found in furniture polish, wood treatment products, coated wooden cutting boards, air fresheners, bathroom cleaners, and kitchen cleaning products, as well as many makeup products, personal-care products, lotions, pharmaceuticals, and automotive products, it may also be used as an ingredient in processed human food products or animal feed. Mineral oil is not readily biodegradable, and it does not come from a renewable resource. There are studies and scientific research that indicate it may compromise immune function.

Triclosan, aka 5-Chloro-2-(2,4-dichlorophenosy)phenol. This chemical is most commonly used as an antibacterial, but it is also used in fabric softeners, disinfectants, trash bags, sink mats, wipes, hand soaps, brooms, mops, sponges, and almost anything marked or labeled "eco-friendly" or "anti-bacterial." You might find it in certain facial-care products. It has been shown to suppress immune function.

Triethanolamine compounds, DEA, TEA, cocomide MEA, DEA-cetyl phosphate, and linoleamide MEA are among a few of the chemicals linked to liver cancer but which are considered to be GRAS. These chemicals are thought to accumulate in the body over time and lead to other types of cancer.

BHT/PHA. Packaged foods, processed foods, plastics, foams, and cosmetics use BHT and BHA (butylated hydroxytoluene and butylated hydroxyanisole), which are synthetic antioxidants found in so many products as preservatives. Their uses range from packaged foods—chips, crackers, cookies—to cosmetics and personal care products. BHT is used in the making of polyurethane foams in furniture and bedding to keep them from turning colors after production and/or catching on fire. It is toluene based and poses a real threat to the normal functioning of the endocrine system, reproductive health, and the organ system. Personal-care products that commonly contain BHA and BHT include fragrances, antiperspirants, makeup, sunscreen, lotions, creams, hair products, and lip moisturizers. Preliminary research of this substance is pointing to a carcinogenic impact.

Flame retardants are used in the manufacturing processes of products used in the furniture, bedding, plastics, and other industries that bring us the comforts of modern civilization. These include polybrominated diphenyl ethers (PDBEs), polybrominated biphenyl (PBB), and brominated cyclohydrocarbons. These are added to many products to prohibit combustion. As we use these products in our preparation of foods (such as plastic cooking utensils) and personal care products and have them in our homes, the possibilities of exposure and associated accumulative immune-suppressive effects increase.

Artificial and synthetic colors and flavors found in all packaged and processed foods are of concern. Of specific interest are the food items marketed specifically to children: cookies, cereals, candy, and chips. Yellow #6, Red #40,

Yellow #5, Blue #1, to name a few, are among the colors used in candy and cereals that are artificially created in a laboratory and have been linked to various central nervous system and neurotoxic irregularities in children and adults. High fructose corn syrup (typically produced from genetically engineered sources) usually leads the ingredient list followed by all the other fun colors and additives. One candy bar typically has more sugar than three donuts and likely contains palm kernel oil, genetically engineered soy lecithin, and toxic saturated fats to compound the problem. You may think "natural flavors" escape scrutiny in the Misner Plan; however, they are typically chemicals that mimic natural flavors and not natural substances imparting that flavor to the food product at all, so we exclude them as much as possible in our diet, as well.

Nail polish historically has used toluene and toluene derivatives since its emergence in the cosmetics market. Salon and nail techs are required to wear protective masks due to the presence of toluene in the nail polish and artificial nail products. Toluene is a known carcinogen and should be avoided completely. Many nail polish manufacturers are now removing toluene from their products, but be sure to read the ingredients carefully to be sure it is not lurking in your favorites. As new products are unveiled at the nail salon, such as dipping powders to replace acrylic nails, and gel polish activated by the known-carcinogenic ultraviolet blue light activator, we encourage you to be aware of the cancer risks associated with these products.

Ethyloxylated ingredients, polyethylene glycols, polysorbates, and dioxanes. Look for ingredients such as laureth, ceteareth, and ceteth in the name, as well as the suffix -sorbates. These indicate that 1,4 dioxane and ethylene oxide are present. These ingredients carry concern for cancer-causing and endocrine-disrupting potential. Found in makeup and cosmetics of various types, it can be tricky to locate them in the ingredient lists of cosmetics, because they have so many other names or monikers. You can search the specific ingredients in your products online if you are unsure.

Fragrances are most often the highest of offenders to those who have liver toxicity, adrenal fatigue syndrome, and other inflammatory diseases, of which cancer is one. This is because of the disruption they cause endocrine system. They are typically simply listed as "natural fragrance," "organic fragrance," or "parfum" in many products, and the individual constituents are not listed. We stay away from any of these ingredients, preferring products that contain organic essential oils.

Fabric softeners and dryer sheets are extremely damaging to the body as they often contain known carcinogens, such as benzyl acetate, alpha terpineol, ethanol (ethyl alcohol), limonene, and chloroform, just to name a few. These chemicals are linked to pancreatic cancer, thyroid problems, and other endocrine disruptions, upper respiratory tract irritants, central nervous system disorders, carcinogens, neurotoxins, and more. Fabric softeners are formulated to coat the fibers of materials and therefore linger on our clothes, where they remain to be inhaled, absorbed, and passively ingested through the respiratory tract and the skin. *Scientific American* and WagWalking.com both report that the just-from-the-dryer freshness you smell from your laundered clothes can cause some serious health problems for you and for your pets. Dryer sheets can be toxic, and even deadly, to cats and dogs as they are cationic (reactant) to the skin, kidney, liver, digestive system, and respiratory system of pets.

Sunscreens contain parabens or aromatic ketones such as oxybenzone, along with other chemicals of concern, such as octinoxate and homosalate. These not only block UV rays of the sun but also disrupt endocrine function and have been suspected of other undesirable accumulative effects on the body's organ systems. Parabens are fairly easy to identify as their name ends in the suffix -paraben. There are more than eighteen parabens used in cosmetics and personal care products. Also present in many sunscreens and cosmetic products is retinyl palmitate (aka Retin-A). Prolonged exposure to retinyl palmitate has been suspected to increase risk of malignant melanoma and disruption of estrogen cycles.

Perflourinated and polytetraflouroethylene compounds (PTFE) are suspected to accumulate in biological systems and adversely affect endocrine function. PTFE compounds have many uses in many industries and are particularly well known as the coatings on non-stick cookware items.

Talc (talcum powder) has recently been proven to be linked to ovarian cancer by the International Agency for Research on Cancer when used on the perineum. When inhaled, talc can irritate the lungs and respiratory system.

Heavy metals are substances that are chemically classified as metals due to their chemical properties. They are commonly present in the earth and are found naturally in many substances and compounds as contaminants. The list of possible contaminants includes cadmium, chromium, lead, nickel, mercury, antimony, and arsenic. In certain dosages and with prolonged exposure by ingestion, inhalation, and absorption, serious accumulative negative effects have been seen in humans. These effects can include irritation, endocrine disruption, reproductive problems, teratogenic (damage in development of embryo or fetus), mutagenic (damage to DNA of an organism), and other types of carcinogenic effects.

BPA (bis-phenol acetone). Considered a xenoestrogen, BPA is a common organic chemical used in the manufacturing of plastics and is a danger to humans because of its ability to masquerade as estrogen in the body. Since our culture uses billions of tons of plastics each year, it is not surprising that the Environmental Working Group (EWG) has compiled data on over 16,000 packaged foods with this hormone-disrupting culprit. BPA may be hiding in aerosol cans, beverage cans, coffee cans, glass bottles and lids, and canned foods. According to the US Centers for Disease Control and Prevention detectable levels of BPA were found in 93% of urine samples taken in 2003-2004 from people six years and older.

We are starting, as consumers, to see ever more labels exclaiming "BPA free" on our plastic containers and bottled waters, as well as some canned items. The

170

Misner Plan recommends avoiding food and drinks that come in contact with plastics. BPA is stable at room temperature but becomes unstable when heated, so if those containers are in the sun (on trucks or in containers during the shipping process) or have hot food put into them, in the case of canned foods, the food or drink item is going to contain this endocrine disrupter. The BPA-free label is also misleading since the new chemical being used to replace BPA has not yet been studied or tested adequately to determine whether it is safe or perhaps even more toxic than BPA. It is allowed to be used until such time as it can be shown to be detrimental to our health. That is not an experiment we personally want to participate in.

You may be surprised, like we were, to learn that chlorinated paper products used in home and healthcare have been treated with BPA after chlorination in order to make them absorbent. This includes toilet paper, paper towels, paper napkins, and facial tissue. To avoid exposure to BPAs in these products, look for the unchlorinated versions that are labeled TCF (totally chlorine free), use cloth napkins, switch to old-fashioned hankies, and when possible, use a bidet for personal cleansing or consider installing an automatic washlet toilet.

Dioxins and polychlorinated biphenyls (PCBs) are directly linked to various cancers. Dioxins such as 1,4 dioxin are present in almost all substances at this time in our lives. You may more readily identify with a pesticide called Agent Orange, which is a dioxin developed in the 1940s and used in the Vietnam War. Dioxins are un-affectionately called the "gift that keeps on giving" because they do not readily degrade, and they are stored in the body's fatty tissues. This is problematic for humans since our brain is nearly 60% fatty tissue. Dioxins can be found in herbicides (weed killers) and pesticides (insect killers and commercial extermination products), but they are also commonly present in the environment as by-products of modern industrial production processes.

Phthalates are chemical groups that are used in almost everything not naturally occurring, including furniture, bedding, construction supplies, detergents, food packaging, personal consumer products, and the list goes on. It is nearly impossible to avoid phthalates because, to put it simply, they have made life easier for all of us within the innovation and convenience of modern culture. Phthalates are easily absorbed through the skin into the bloodstream and are found in vinyl products, plastics, food packaging, medication and medical devices, baby formula, pesticides, wallpaper, scented products such as air fresheners, perfumes, colognes, aftershaves, scented candles, electronics, toys, and jewelry.

Atrazine is an herbicide typically used against grasses and weeds but which is also widely used on crops of corn, sugarcane, pineapple, and sorghum. Recently it has been found in our public drinking water. It has been found linked to low fetal weight and heart, urinary, and limb defects in infants when the mother was exposed to it. A water filter certified to remove atrazine will remove much of the atrazine from your household water supply, and your produce should be washed thoroughly and come from organic sources, and even then washed thoroughly all the same. We recommend using a whole-house filtration system that includes several chambers (including UV light), and then finish off your drinking water with a reverse osmosis system under the sink. This allows both solid contaminant particles and dissolved solids to be filtered out so that your drinking and cooking water is as pure as possible. This water will not be alkaline, so adding either lemon or trace minerals to the water before drinking it will be necessary.

Organophosphates are found in pesticides and herbicides, particularly in flea and tick medications for your household pets. Along with atrazine and organophosphates in the meat and produce we eat and the water we drink, perchlorate is another offender found in the public drinking water and is unavoidable. Again, an adequate water filtration system is needed. Check the EWG's list of water filtration systems to select the best one for your home.

Glycol ethers (polyether glycols) and 2-butoxyethanol (EGBE) and methoxydiglycol (DEGME) have been linked to shrunken testicles in male rats exposed to glycol ethers, which have also been shown to lead to respiratory problems, such as asthma, allergies, and blood abnormalities by the EWG. These are found in paint, paint thinners, solvents, and other construction materials. Polyethylene glycols (PEG) are also found in skin care, hair care, and other personal care products. Remember that if it goes on your skin, it goes into your blood stream.

So, now that you know what we have learned about these ingredients, you may never look at things like laundry soap, facial wash, and even toilet paper the same again. We hope not. We hope that at this point you are asking, "But what are we supposed to do?" Fortunately, most stores offer scent-free, organic alternatives to cleaning products that have a high toxic burden, including the simple "soap nut" which we've been using for a few years now. You can also use wool balls in your dryer instead of the problematic dryer sheets. You also have non-toxic options for dish soap, but watch the ingredients list to be sure there isn't something objectionable hiding in the "all-natural" product that looks good from the front of the bottle. Read the small print!

For other products, we have included in part three of this book a section of recipes, so you can make your own facial cleanser, body cream, and even toothpaste right out of your kitchen. Remember, that if you cannot eat it, you do not want it on your skin! We have also included some recommended lines of skin care, makeup, and hair care products in our resource section. Our list is not meant to be exhaustive, but it will get you going in the right direction for abundant health.

And since we will never be able to completely eliminate environmental toxins and endocrine disrupters from our lives, we hope you will join us in the Misner Plan to eat so well that your body is supported in its natural ability to detoxify.

Common Sources of Endocrine Disrupting Chemicals

These substances listed below have been known to be used in the production processes associated with the products listed at one time. This list is not exclusive or comprehensive.

Antiperspirants/Deodorants

aluminum

fragrance

talc

Cosmetics

talc

retinol

retinyl palmitate

mineral oil

formaldehyde,

quaternium-15,

imidazolidinyl urea

toluene

alpha hydroxy acids

glycolic acid

phthalates

paraben

Dental Care Products

PTFE (dental floss)

amalgam fillings (mercury)

bleach (root canals)

Dry Cleaning Solvents/Laundry Detergents

1, 1 trichloroethane

perchloroethane

sodium lauryl sulfate

Fabric Softeners/Dryer Sheets

benzyl acetate

alpha terpineol

ethyl alcohol

chloroform

limonene

Food & Water Supply

bisphenol A

vinclozolin (antifungal)

polycarbonate plastic (food can liners)

phthalates

antibiotics

atrazine

arsenic

perchlorate

heavy metals (fish and seafood)

antibiotics & hormones in meats & dairy

soy & beta sitosterol in foods

Furniture/Bedding/Flooring

formaldehyde

BHT

BHA

Household Products

PTFE

PFCs

BPA

PFOA

fire retardants (clothing, furniture, flooring materials)

PVC (polyvinylchloride) plastic bath toys

heavy metals (mercury, lead, cadmium, chromium) paint

thinners/solvents

organophosphates

triclosan (antimicrobials)

ethylene glycols

1,1 trichlorbenzene (stain removers)

ammonia (glass cleaner)

bleach

paraffins, limonene (furniture polish)

Lotions/Cremes/ Moisturizers

fragrances (unidentified)

DEA, TEA

cocomide

Mouthwashes/Oral Rinses

chlorhexidine

thymol

gluconate

cetylpyridinium chloride

triclosan

Nail Polish

formaldehyde

heavy metals (lead, cadmium)

phthalates

chloroform

acetone (polish remover)

acrylic (artificial nail powder)

Paint/Paint Thinners/Glues/Solvents

formaldehyde

heavy metals

organophosphates

glycol ethers

triclocarban

lead

Pesticides/Herbicides/Agricultural Chemicals

chlorpyrifos (pesticide)

methoxychlor (pesticide)

dichlorodiphenyltrichloroethane (DDT) (pesticide)

tributyltin (pesticide)

Pharmaceuticals

hormone replacement therapy

oral contraceptives

diethylstilbestrol

Plastics (Containers/Bags/Misc.)

phthalates (PVC, vinyl products, plastic wrap, fragrances)

Soap/Shampoos/Hand Sanitizers

sodium lauryl sulfate

triclosan (antimicrobial)

selenium sulfide

1,4 dioxane

bronopol

Sunscreens

oxybenzene

benzylalkonium

octinoxate

homosalate

parabens

Miscellaneous

non-stick coatings and cookware (PTFE)

office products (ink, toner, solvents)

thermal papers from cash register receipts

currency (various contaminants)

stain resistant clothing (PFCs)

feminine hygiene products

adult diapers (phthalates, plastics)

PART THREE:
HEALTHY SKIN CARE RECIPES

Love is the Healer
By Beth Misner

While on this healing journey,
I take as my closest companion—LOVE.

I breathe in white light, and
I breathe out all the energy I don't need.
I inhale peace, calm, and equanimity;
I exhale hurry, worry, and stress.

My healing includes love and laughter.
There are some things doctors can do,
While there are other things only I can do,
Like relax, rest, and enjoy every moment of life.

Nature is all around me.
I smile as birdsong fills the air.
The quiet sound of the waterfall—
Perfect accompaniment for their voices.

With a full and joyous heart,
I sit quietly, knowing that
I am in the Universe, and the Universe
Is in my body—we are combined as one.

"The cellular transformation
Is vibrant and complete
Into wholeness and perfection."

HEALING CAN BE EASY

While on this healing journey,
I take as my closest companion—LOVE.
And I am healed, completely healed.

I embrace this reality.
I embrace this truth.

And so it is.

FACIAL TREATMENT

Dr. Mohammad Nikkhah

This treatment is derived from a facial ritual used by Cleopatra. Since our modern facial products, which are laden with chemicals and preservatives, were not available to her, she was known for her elaborate bathing and skin-care rituals composed from natural ingredients found in the kitchen and fields around her.

Set aside plenty of time, about 30 minutes, for this wonderful facial treatment, and indulge your skin in a ritual that has been handed down through many generations. You'll be amazed at how great your skin will look and feel. Soon your friends will be asking you what product line you switched to.

Ingredients and Supplies

10-12 clean washcloths (unbleached, organic cotton)

Makeup pads (unbleached, organic cotton)

1 lemon or lime, sliced into about 14 rings (enough to cover the face)

4-5 oz full-fat milk (goat milk preferred) in small bowl

1 cucumber, sliced into 20 rings (enough to cover the face)

1 medium aloe vera leaf

Plastic knife

15-20 oz very warm water in bowl

15-20 oz ice water (use plenty of ice) in bowl

15-20 oz hot chamomile tea in bowl

Timer

Instructions

Step 1: Clean your face of all makeup and remove jewelry, including earrings.

Step 2: Using warm water from the first bowl, make a compress with a clean washcloth and apply to the face for 30-60 seconds. This will serve to open the pores and prepare the skin to absorb the nutrients in the ingredients used in the facial treatment.

Step 3: Lie comfortably and place as many slices of the lemon or lime on the face as will fit. Make sure to avoid the eye area. Close your eyes and rest for five minutes. Any remaining debris on the skin will begin to break down, and Vitamin C will be administered to the facial tissues. After five minutes, remove the citrus and discard slices. Wipe your face clean with a washcloth soaked in warm water to remove the remnants of the citrus fruit.

Step 4: Using a cotton makeup pad, apply milk to the face until the skin is saturated. Milk provides nourishment and healthy fats to the epithelial layers of the skin. Leave the milk on your skin for five minutes. Then, wipe the face clean with a washcloth soaked in warm water to remove the remnants of the milk.

Step 5: Do five consecutive chamomile tea compresses. Each compress lasts for 15 seconds. I have found it helpful to have all five washcloths in the bowl of hot tea in order to be able to quickly apply each new compress. Caution: Be sure to wring out the washcloths of excess liquid and make sure it is not too hot before applying to your face. Then, use a clean washcloth to pat the face dry. You will find that the chamomile tea relaxes both you and your face.

Step 6: Following the chamomile tea compresses, lie back again, and apply the cucumber slices all over the face. Cucumber hydrates and conditions your facial tissues to receive more hydration. Close your eyes and place cucumber slices on each eyelid. Relax for five minutes. Remove the cucumber slices and discard.

Step 7: Open the aloe vera leaf with the plastic knife. Scrape out the gel and apply directly to your face using either your hands or a cotton makeup pad. Before you lie back and rest, submerge a clean washcloth in the bowl with the ice water (to be used in the last step of this facial treatment). Then rest for five minutes, allowing the aloe vera to dry. Aloe vera will deeply hydrate your skin. After five minutes, remove the aloe vera gel with a clean washcloth soaked in warm water.

Step 8: Finally, apply the chilled compress to your face. Leave this compress in place for 20 seconds or the amount of time you are comfortable with it. This final step will close your pores to allow your skin to retain all the moisture and nutrients you just infused into it.

NATURAL DEODORANT
AND TOOTHPASTE

Ingredients

⅛ cup organic coconut oil, softened

1 Tbsp baking soda

2 drops essential oil of your choice (optional)

Instructions

Combine ingredients in a small bowl until completely mixed, then transfer to a small storage jar or 2-ounce condiment cup with lid.

To apply, scoop out a small amount (about the size of a pea) and apply to underarms. You will still perspire, but the baking soda will be absorbent, and the coconut oil will kill bacteria, keeping you comfortably fresh all day long.

To create toothpaste from these ingredients, use peppermint, spearmint, or orange essential oil. Brush twice per day, swishing the paste around your mouth before rinsing with warm water. Your gums and teeth will thank you.

GENTLE FACIAL CLEANSER

Ingredients

⅓ cup organic almond oil

1 tsp castor oil

Instructions

Mix two oils together in a small jar and store in your bathroom cabinet.

To use, dampen your face with warm water, smooth cleanser onto face, and remove with a warm, soft washcloth. Pat face dry.

GREEN GODDESS FACE MASK

Ingredients

¼ organic avocado, mashed

1 tsp organic sesame oil

1 tsp raw local honey

2 drops lemon essential oil

Instructions

Combine ingredients in a small bowl with a wooden spoon until creamy and smooth.

Scoop into your palm and smooth evenly onto your damp face and neck. Let mask sit on your skin for about 10 minutes.

Rinse face thoroughly with warm water and pat dry.

RUBY RED GRAPEFRUIT
FACIAL TONER

Ingredients

3 cups water

¼ tsp raw local honey

½ grapefruit peel, cut into strips

Instructions

Bring water to barely a simmer, and then set aside and allow to cool slightly.

Stir honey into warm water until dissolved.

Add grapefruit peel strips to ½ quart jar and cover with honey water. Allow to stand for two to three hours.

Strain the water into a spritz bottle for use. Honey is anti-bacterial and anti-fungal, so it serves as a natural preservative for your toner.

Tip: This toner will feel even better to your skin if you refrigerate it and apply cold.

CHAMOMILE AND MINT TONER

Ingredients

   1 cup of water

   1 Tbsp dried chamomile flowers

   1 tsp dried mint leaves

Instructions

Boil the water and infuse with the dried chamomile flowers and mint leaves.

Let steep for 15 minutes, covered, then strain and allow to cool.

Pour into storage jar and apply daily with an unbleached, organic cotton pad after cleansing.

WHIPPED BODY CREAM

Ingredients

1 cup organic coconut oil, softened (not runny)

1 tsp organic grape seed oil

10 drops of essential oil of choice

Instructions

Combine ingredients and use an immersion blending stick to blend until frothy.

Pour into a small glass storage container or into a short, fat jar. Store in a cool spot close to where you will want to use it.

When you are ready to use it, soften by placing jar in a bowl of hot water, and let your skin love the healing properties of this healthy cream.

You can also use this body cream for shaving.

NATURAL HAIR CARE

Clarifying and Balancing Shampoo

Ingredients

    1 cup hot water

    2 tsp apple cider vinegar

    1 Tbsp baking soda

Instructions

Combine ingredients and stir. Allow to cool, then transfer to a squeeze bottle.

Use daily in order to clean scalp and hair.

Creamy Conditioner

Ingredient

    Plain yogurt

Instructions

Apply ⅛ to ¼ cup of yogurt to wet hair, and leave in for 20 minutes. Rinse thoroughly.

Curly Hair Boost

Ingredients

1 cup water

½ tsp sea salt

3 drops essential oil of choice

Instructions

Stir salt into water until dissolved, then add essential oil drops. Transfer to small spray bottle.

Spray lightly into damp hair, scrunch and allow to air dry or use a blow dryer diffuser attachment for a beachy, curly look.

Tip: Avoid using this daily, as it may be drying to your hair when used frequently. To freshen your look each day, mist your hair with fresh water to dampen the ends, scrunch again, and allow to air dry or diffuse.

PART FOUR:
RESOURCE SECTION

Henani

By Beth Misner

"Henani," I said to God.
"Here I am."

With that opening
In my heart, my soul,
Came true willingness
To be used by God.

And the response
To my "Henani"
Was
. . .Unmistakable
. . . Unavoidable
. . .Unimaginable.

It was the day
The death of
The egoic self commenced.

HEALTH CLINICS AND
DOCTORS TO INVESTIGATE

Betty Runkle, ND, Texas www.bettyrunkle.com

Center for Advanced Medicine, Southern California
www.centerforadvancedmed.com

Clínica CIPAG, Dr. Isai Castillo, Baja California www.drcastillo.com

Eden Valley Institute of Wellness, Colorado http://www.eden-valley.org/

Hufeland Klinik, Germany www.hufeland.com

Issels Medical Center, Central California www.issels.com

Kevin Kelly, MD, Southern California www.kevinkellymd.com

Sean Stringer, DC, DIM, DMM, MO, Florida www.bodyminddoc.com

READING MATERIAL

Cancer: A Second Opinion by Dr. Josef Issels

Cancer: Step Outside the Box by Ty Bollinger

Conversation with the Heart by Lise Janelle, DC

The Genie in Your Genes by Dawson Church

Head to Toe Healing by Chunyi Lin

Heal Breast Cancer Naturally: 7 Essential Steps to Beating Breast Cancer by Dr. Veronique Desaulniers

Love, Medicine, and Miracles by Bernie Siegel

You Are the Placebo by Joe Dispenza

NATURAL PRODUCTS

Adaptogens and Nervines www.bettyrunkle.com

Beta Glucans: Sacred 7 Mushroom Extract Powder www.naturealmco.com

CBD Oil, Organic/High Potency www.legendshealth.net

Chemical-free Laundry Soap www.econutssoap.com

Chemical-free and Edible Skin Care www.annmariegianni.com

King of Coffee https://seansmiley.myorganogold.com

Lentin 1000 Plus www.lentinplus.com.my

Misner Plan www.misnerplan.com

Organic Essential Oils www.rockymountainoils.com

Osage Orange (Hedge Apples) www.Amazon.com (fresh when in season, or freeze-dried, powdered)

Reishi Mushroom Spore Powder, Ganoderma Lucidum
www.seansmiley.myorganogold.com

ACKNOWLEDGEMENTS

First and foremost, I would like to give my heartfelt thanks to my husband, Ivan. Your unwavering support of my choices on the path I walked, which you had already walked before me, meant so much. Your love and tenderness increased every day of this amazing journey. I appreciate you so much. And to all the loving members of my family who never once questioned my decisions or nagged me to do anything other than what I was doing, I want you to know how much I love you all. And finally, all my gratitude goes to my team of doctors and advisors who never let me down along the way to my recovery.

Beth Misner

I'm incredibly thankful for Beth's strength, resolve, and determination to heal. The grace and dignity with which you approached this challenging situation was inspiring. I thought I had done pretty well using the mind-body connection to bring about my own healing, but you really took it to a whole higher level. I am also grateful to the team of physicians and experts who guided Beth, encouraging her and empowering her to take a natural approach to healing.

Ivan Misner, Ph.D.

I would like to acknowledge my husband, Robert, whose logical, consistent, and steady thinking always brings me back to center and whose support has been the absolute foundation of all my successes. To my four children, Ryan, Garrett,

Jensyn, and Evan, who are the world's best "test subjects," I would like to say that you are my greatest accomplishments. Special thanks to my dear friends, Alan and the late Cynthia Reed (1956-2016) for your mentorship, your constant loving support, and your belief in my dream of serving others through health education. I love you all so dearly.

Betty Wells Runkle, N.D.

I owe my success to God, my parents Ashraf Beyzaei and Bagher Nikkhah, my wife Mahtab Nikkhah, and my two sons Arash and Afsheen Nikkhah. Without their help and sacrifice, I would not have been able to accomplish what I have.

Dr. Mohammad Nikkhah

ABOUT THE AUTHORS

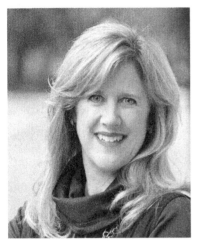

CoAuthor Beth Misner has been involved in functional healthcare in one aspect or another since her early 20s when she worked as a chiropractic assistant. She currently holds a certification in sports nutrition and is working on her Medical Qigong Practitioner certification. She is a black belt in karate and teaches t'ai chi chuan, qigong, and meditation. Her two previous books, *Jesus and the Secret* and *Healing Begins in the Kitchen*, offer more insight into her approach to life best lived with an understanding of the interconnection of the BodyMind. Websites: www.BethMisner.com and www.MisnerPlan.com.

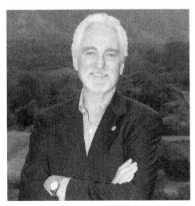

CoAuthor Ivan Misner, PhD, is the founder and chief visionary officer of BNI. He is a *New York Times* best-selling author, entrepreneur, and the cofounder of the BNI Foundation and Asentiv. His drive and initiative have touched many people all over the globe with his Givers Gain attitude. His previous experience of healing cancer naturally, without conventional treatments, prepared him to support his wife, Beth, on her own path of using alternative healthcare to move into wellness. Websites: www.IvanMisner.com and www.MisnerPlan.com.

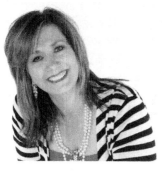

CoAuthor Betty Wells Runkle, ND, is a traditional naturopath and member of the Certified Natural Health Professionals Association. Betty has an AS in natural science and her bachelor's studies were done at Texas A&M University with a major in microbiology and immunology. Although her early career started in the field of analytical chemistry, her passion for people and for science drove her eventually to seek nutritional and herbal education so that she could better influence and empower others. Website: www.BettyRunkle.com

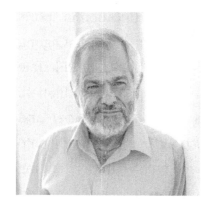

Contributing Author Dr. Mohammad Nikkhah, is a gifted holistic practitioner and healer. With a background in healing practices from the Middle East, China, and India, as well as Native American medical traditions, he has an understanding of the systems of the body that few doctors ever achieve. Directing the focus of his practice to include energy work, herbs, and nutrition has allowed him to facilitate healing for his patients from an integrated approach. He has traveled the world over, both learning and helping others find wellness by working with the body's innate systems.

INDEX

Atrazine, 172
Autologous
 Cytokine, 37, 71
 Dendritic Cells, 31, 37
 Lymphokine-Activated Killer (LAK) Cells, 30, 33
Ayurveda, 44, 153-4, 160

B

B17 *See* Laetrile
Baby
 Formula, 172
 Soap, 166
Bacteria, 140, 160, 182
Baking Soda, 182, 188
Balance, 147-8
Barley, 116
Barnes, Samuel, 74
Barnett, 138
Beard, John (Dr.), 136
Bedding, 167, 171, 175
Benzyl Acetate, 169, 174
Benzylalkonium, 176
Beta Glucan, 115-6, 127, 194
Beta Sitosterol, 175
Bettyrunkle.Com, 192, 194
Big Red Tea Cup Bird Feeder, 34, 125
Bio-Accumulation, 164
Biobran *See* MGN-3
Biopsy, 5, 11-9, 26, 32-, 107-8, 110
Bis-Phenol Acetone (BPA), 163, 170-1, 175
Bisphenol A, 174
Bitter Almond Oil, 141, 146
Blackmore, 138
Bleach, 174-5
Blood
 Abnormalities, 173
 Alkalinity, 123
 Biopsy, 33, 107
 Sugar, 48
Body
 Adaptogens, 159
 And Absorption, 118
Bodyminddoc.Com, 192
Bone Marrow, 116, 162
Bowel Function, 113, 127

Breast Scans (Bi-Rads), 18, 24, 26, 33, 108
Broccoli, 129, 133, 140, 145
Brominated Cyclohydrocarbons, 167
Bromopol, 165
Bronopol, 176
Brussels Sprouts, 133, 140
Bujo, 71-2
Butylated Hydroxyanisole (BHA), 167, 175
Butylated Hydroxytoluene (BHT), 167, 175

C

C-Reactive Protein (CRP), 135
Cadmium, 170
Calcium D-Glucarate, 140
Cancer
 Cells, 34-6, 76, 138
  Anaerobic Environment, 132
  Relaxation, 143
  See Melatonin
  Weakening Of, 129-30, 132, 137, 143
  Gastric, 139
 Of Breast, 2, 3, 5, 12, 17, 18, 32-3, 83, 92, 97-8, 138
 Prostate, 4, 11, 17-9, 23, 108, 125, 165
 See Also Vitamin D3
 Stem Cell (CSC), 26, 33
Cancer Healing Meditation, 39
Cabernet Sauvignon, 97
Caffeine, 56
Caisse, Renée, 142
Calcium, 123, 140, 145
Canada, 166
Carbohydrates, 42, 62, 135-6
Carcinogen, 44, 47, 114-5, 121, 164, 168-9
Carcinoma, 29
Carotenoids, 158
Cassava Plant
Cauliflower, 133, 140-1
CBD, 141, 146, 194
Cefestol, 114
Center for Advanced Medicine, 10
Central Nervous System, 156-7, 162, 168-9
Ceteareth, 168
Ceteth, 168
Cetylpyridinium Chloride, 175

Made in the USA
Columbia, SC
20 July 2019